How to Use This Book

This book serves two different functions. It can either be used as a dictionary of immunology or as a concise revision guide/study aid. Readers who already know some immunology and require a summary of particular aspects, should consult the contents page. The book is divided into seven chapters each of which contains a number of related topics.

To use the book as a dictionary, look up the word or abbreviation in the Index of Terms (pages ix to xxv). This gives a single page number where a definition of the word will be found - associated words will be found on the same page. Page references to particular topics set out on several pages are indicated in bold figures.

Acknowledgements

I am most grateful to my coeditors, Professor Ivan Roitt and Dr Jonathan Brostoff for letting me use or adapt some of the illustrations which previously appeared in our book 'Immunology'. I would like to thank the contributors who inspired those diagrams, including Drs Frank Hay, Peter Lydyard, Anne Cooke, Graham Rook, Micheal Owen, Roger Taylor, Marc Feldmann, Michael Crumpton, James Howard, Malcolm Turner and Professor Michael Steward. In addition, Fig. 1.1 (mast cell) appears by courtesy of Dr. B. Greenwood, Fig. 5.6 by courtesy of Professor C.H.W. Horne and Fig. 7.8 by courtesy of Dr B. Dean. Naturally a book of this kind cannot include everything of interest to immunologists; I have tried to cover all the essential areas of the subject, but I should be pleased to know when the readers consider that particular subjects deserve further detail.

Contents

1 THE IMMUNE SYSTEM

2 ANTIBODIES AND ANTIGEN

3 THE IMMUNE RESPONSE

IMMUNOLOGY

An Illustrated Outline

IMMUNOLOGY

An Illustrated Outline

DAVID MALE MA PhD

Lecturer in Neuroimmunology
Institute of Psychiatry
London SE5

Churchill Livingstone
Edinburgh • London • Melbourne • New York

Gower Medical Publishing • London • New York • 1986

Distributors of English Editions

World except USA, Canada, Mexico and Japan

Churchill Livingstone
Medical Division of Longman Group Limited,
Robert Stevenson House, 1-3 Baxter's Place,
Leith Walk, Edinburgh EH1 3AF

USA, Canada and Mexico

The C.V. Mosby Company
11830 Westline Industrial Drive, St. Louis,
Missouri 63146

Project Editor   David Bennett
Designer   Celia Welcomme
Line Artist   Karen Cochrane

Printed in Great Britain by Hazell Watson & Viney Ltd.

Typeset by Informat

British Library Cataloguing in Publication Data
Male, D.K.
   Immunology: An Illustrated Outline.
   1. Immunology
   I. Title
   616.07'9   QR181

ISBN 0443-037-639 (Churchill Livingstone)
      0-906923-58-1 (Gower)

4 HISTOCOMPATIBILITY LOCI AND TRANSPLANTATION

5 INFLAMMATION AND PHAGOCYTOSIS

6 IMMUNOPATHOLOGY

7 IMMUNOLOGICAL TESTS AND TECHNIQUES

Index of Terms

Bold numbers indicate that a section is devoted to that term.
Italic numbers indicate that the term is included in a table.

A

D

I

Q

1 The Immune System

INTRODUCTION

The function of the immune system is to protect the body from damage caused by invading microorganisms - bacteria, viruses, fungi and parasites. This defensive function is performed by the leucocytes (white blood cells) and a number of accessory cells, which are distributed throughout the organs of the body, but tend to cluster in a number of lymphoid organs, including the bone marrow, thymus, spleen and lymph nodes. Accumulations of these cells are also found in tissues where pathogens might enter the body, such as the mucosa of the gut and lung. The various cells interact with each other producing a coordinated immune response directed towards eliminating the pathogen or minimizing the damage it causes.

Lymphocytes are the key cells controlling the immune response. They specifically recognize 'foreign' material and distinguish it from the body's own components. Generally they react to the foreign material but not against the body's tissue. Lymphocytes are of two main types: B cells which produce antibodies, and T cells which have a number of functions including 1) helping B cells to make antibody, 2) recognizing and destroying cells infected with virus, 3) activating phagocytes to destroy the pathogens they have taken up, and 4) controlling the level and quality of the immune response. Lymphocytes recognize foreign material by specific surface receptor molecules (antigen receptor). To specifically recognize the enormous variety of different molecules, the antigen receptors must be equally diverse. During lymphocyte development recombination and rearrangement of the antigen receptor genes occurs, so that the lymphocyte population as a whole has a great diversity of antigen receptors, although any one lymphocyte can only make one type of receptor and thus recognizes only a very limited number of antigens.

Phagocytes include blood monocytes, macrophages and neutrophils. Their function is to take up pathogens, foreign material and cell debris and to break it down. Macrophages also transport antigen to lymph nodes where it stimulates lymphocytes. Antibodies (secreted by B cells) bound to particles allow them to be recognized by the phagocytes.

1

Accessory cells include eosinophil and basophil granulocytes, mast cells, platelets and antigen-presenting cells. Eosinophils have a role in damaging parasites and controlling inflammation. Basophils, mast cells and platelets contain a variety of molecules which mediate inflammation. They are thus important in linking immune responses and inflammatory reactions. Antigen-presenting cells include several cell types which present antigen to lymphocytes. All these cell types react in a coordinated way to produce an effective immune response.

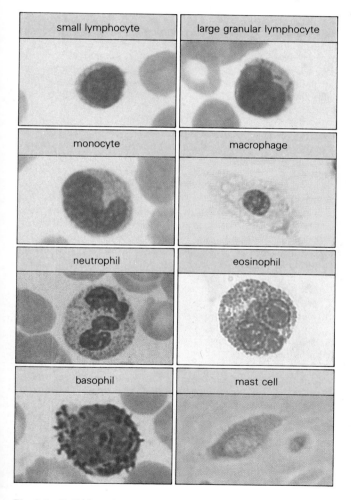

Fig.1.1 Cells involved in the immune response.

LYMPHOCYTES

B cells are lymphocytes which develop in foetal liver and subsequently in bone marrow. Birds have a specialized organ, the bursa of Fabricius, in which B cells develop. Mature B cells carry surface immunoglobulin which acts as their antigen receptor. They then move through the circulation to secondary lymphoid tissues, where they respond to antigenic stimuli by dividing and differentiating into plasma cells under the control of lymphokines released by T cells.

Plasma cells / Antibody forming cells (AFCs) are terminally differentiated B cells. They have an expanded cytoplasm with characteristic parallel arrays of rough endoplasmic reticulum and are entirely devoted to the production of secreted antibody. Plasma cells are seen in the red pulp of the spleen, the medulla of lymph nodes, the MALT and in small numbers at sites of inflammation.

T cells are lymphocytes which develop in the thymus. This organ is seeded during embryonic development by lymphocyte stem cells from the bone marrow. Immature T cells occupy the thymic cortex, while more mature cells are seen in the medulla. There is considerable T cell proliferation and cell death within the thymus, such that the majority of developing T cells die before leaving this organ. T cells acquire their antigen receptors in the thymus and differentiate into a number of subpopulations which have separate functions, and which can be recognized by their different cell surface molecules (markers). The subpopulations are.

T helper (T_H) cells. These T lymphocytes help B cells to produce antibody. To make antibody to most antigens (T-dependent antigens), it is necessary that both T and B cells recognize different parts of the antigen. T helper cells also cooperate with cytotoxic T cells in the recognition of allogeneic grafts and virally-infected cells. They also release lymphokines which can activate macrophages and other cell types. T helper cells recognize antigen in association with class 2 molecules encoded by the major histocompatibility complex (MHC).

T inducer cells is a term used to describe the activity of T helper cells in activating other types of T cells.

T delayed hypersensitivity (T_D) cells are the T cells responsible for bringing macrophages and other inflammatory cells to areas where delayed hypersensitivity reactions occur. These T cells are probably a functionally active group of T helper cells rather than a distinct subpopulation.

T cytotoxic (Tc) cells, are capable of destroying allogeneic cells and virally-infected target cells, which they recognize by interaction with antigens and MHC class 1 molecules on the target cell surface.

T suppressor (Ts) cells regulate the action of other T cells and B cells. They may be functionally divided according to whether their suppressive action is specific for cells with particular antigen receptors or non-specific. Their actions are sometimes, but not always MHC restricted.

Memory cells. These are functionally defined lymphocytes which can be either B cells or T cells. They are responsible for the maintenance of specific immunological memory following a primary immune response. Although the idea of memory cells is intellectually useful, there is not, as yet, any specific way of identifying them although it has been suggested that memory B cells have completed a number of their differentiation steps and have little surface IgM.

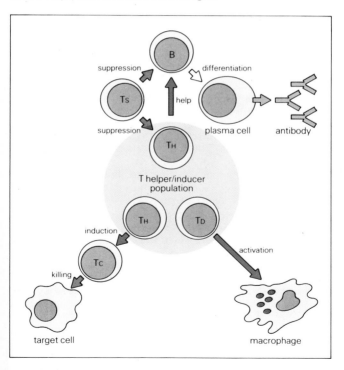

Fig. 1.2   Relations and interactions of lymphocytes.

4

L CELLS / NULL CELLS

L cells / Null (non-T, non-B) cells / Third population cells are all descriptions of a distinct population of leucocytes constituting 14% of blood monocytes. They have properties intermediate between T lymphocytes and myelomonocytic cells. For example, some of these cells possess the T3 T cell marker *and* the OKM1 myeloid cell marker. It appears that the T cell markers are expressed early during their maturation and the myeloid markers develop later. The great majority possess high density Fc receptors which bind IgG strongly at 4°C but weakly at 37°C. The majority of the leucocyte K cell and NK cell activity is found in this population of cells. They also have some regulatory suppressive functions.

Large Granular Lymphocytes (LGL) is a morphological description of a population of lymphocyte like cells containing a large amount of cytoplasm with azurophilic granules. They constitute 5 - 15% of peripheral blood monocytes. This population also contains K cell and NK cell activity. It is thought that LGLs are mature L cells, and 70 - 80% of isolated L cells have LGL morphology.

Tγ cells are blood monocytes with surface Fcγ receptors (ie. for IgG), which may be isolated by rosetting. This population contains a number of cells with T suppressor/cytotoxic markers (T8) but the majority are L cells. They are capable of suppressing antibody synthesis.

Tμ cells are blood lymphocytes with surface Fcμ receptors (ie. for IgM). It has been inferred that these cells can help the antibody response. For example, it has been shown in a number of systems that, whereas the passive administration of antigen-specific IgG suppresses the antibody response, the administration of specific IgM enhances it.

K (Killer) cells are monocytes which can kill target cells sensitized with antibody, which they bind via their Fc receptors; the majority are L cells.

NK (Natural Killer) cells are capable of killing a number of virally-infected and transformed target cells to which they have not been previously sensitized. They have not been separated from K cells, although K cell activity and NK activity develop independently.

Effector and Target cells are functional descriptions applied where any cell type (effector) acts upon another (target), but particularly where the effector kills the target.

5

ANTIGEN RECEPTORS

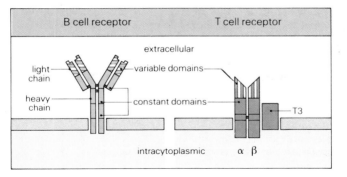

Fig.1.3 Antigen receptors of the B and T cells.

T cells and B cells have different types of antigen receptor, although they both have a common molecular ancestry. The B cell's receptor is a membrane immunoglobulin consisting of two identical pairs of disulphide-linked light and heavy chains. The antigen binding portion is located at the end of the V domains. The T cell receptor is composed of an α and a β chain, each with a variable and a constant domain, which may be associated with the cell surface molecule T3 (in humans) or its equivalent. The genes for the variable (antigen binding) domains are generated by recombination between separate types of gene segment, termed V, D and J. For example, the region encoding the T cell β chain has an undetermined number of V and D segments and two sets of J segments. These can recombine in many different combinations to give a single VDJ gene which encodes the variable domain of the β chain. The VDJ gene is united with the adjoining C region gene to form mRNA (VDJC) which is translated to form a complete β chain.

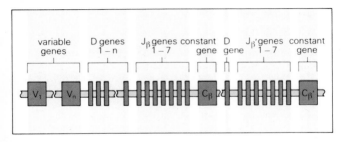

Fig.1.4 Genes of the mouse T cell β chain.

MARKERS

Lymphocytes and other leucocytes are differentiated by their cell surface molecules, identified with specific antibodies, and by their intracytoplasmic enzymes and granule contents. The most readily accessible marker of B cells is the surface immunoglobulin (antigen receptor), but other types of molecules are useful for distinguishing subsets of T cells. Some of the more commonly used markers are listed below. Terminologically the names of monoclonal antibodies used to identify the markers is often also applied to the markers themselves.

Thy (θ) is an allelically variable molecule encoded on mouse chromosome 9, present on all T cells.

Ly (Lyt) antigens. These are a large series of cell surface molecules found on mouse T cells. Only the Ly1, 2 and 3 molecules have so far proved useful in differentiating between the T cells subsets. Thus, Ly1 encoded on chromosome 19 is found on T helper cells; Ly2 and Ly3, encoded by closely linked genes on chromosome 6, occur on cytotoxic and suppressor T cells, and appear to function in MHC class I molecule restricted interactions (cf. T8).

Lyb antigens are surface molecules of mouse B cells. The Lyb5 antigen identifies a subset of B cells which is responsive to a particular group of T independent antigens.

L3T4, present on mouse T helper cells, appears to be linked to MHC class 2 restriction, and is thus equivalent to T4 in man.

CD markers. New designation for human lymphocyte surface protein recognized by antibodies. Some are identical to OKT antigens.

	mouse T cell			human T cell	
all T cells	Thy1			(T1/CD5),T3/CD3,T11/CD2	
T_H, T_D	Ly1	Qa1	L3T4	T4/CD4	T1/CD5
T_S, T_C	Ly2, 3			T8/CD8	
all activated T cells	Ia			HLA-DR	TAC/CD25

Fig.1.5 Summary of the surface markers on mouse and human peripheral T cells.

T (OKT) antigens are human T cell surface markers.

T1(CD5) is present on all T cells and some B cells.

T3(CD3) is a protein involved in cell activation which is associated with the T cell's antigen receptor (Ti).

T4(CD4), present on helper cells, is involved in MHC class 2 restricted interactions.

T6(CD1) is a developmental marker, which is only present on cortical thymocytes and is subsequently lost.

T8(CD8) is present on cytotoxic and suppressor T cells and is involved in MHC class 1 restricted interactions. Some thymocytes have both T4 and T8, but one or other of the markers is lost during differentiation.

TII(CD2) is the receptor which binds sheep erythrocytes and may be involved in antigen non-specific cell activation.

TAC(CD25) is the cell surface receptor for interleukin 2.

OKM1 identifies a glycoprotein on the surface of monocytes, granulocytes and mature L cells.

HNK1 identifies NK (natural killer) cells and so reacts with the majority of L cells.

MAC-1 is a surface antigen on macrophages and NK cells which may be identical to the C3bi receptor, CR3.

α-Naphthyl acid esterase (ANAE) is an enzyme which appears as a few clustered dots on stained T cells (and also on monocytes in a diffuse pattern).

Acid phosphatase is seen in T cells, but also occurs in neutrophils, eosinophils and L cells.

Mitogens are molecules which induce differentiation and division (mitosis) of cells. A few are commonly used by immunologists to induce lymphocyte activation including:

LPS (Lipopolysaccharide) (endotoxin), derived from the cell wall of Gram negative bacteria, is a polyclonal B cell mitogen in mice, and induces immunoglobulin secretion.

PHA (Phytohaemagglutinin) is a T cell mitogen which can also trigger cell functions and lymphokine production.

Con-A (Concanavalin A) is a T cell mitogen which stimulates both primed and unprimed cells.

PWM (Pokeweed mitogen) stimulates both T and B cells, and can induce IgM synthesis by B cells.

ANTIGEN-PRESENTING CELLS

Antigen-presenting cells (APCs). Most antigens must be picked up and transported via the lymphatic system to secondary lymphoid organs (for example, the spleen and lymph nodes) before they are presented to lymphocytes in a form which they can recognize. These functions are performed by phagocytes and/or antigen-presenting cells. Some cells, including some macrophages, are capable of performing both functions. Often, antigen must be processed before lymphocytes can recognize it. For example, T helper cells must 'see' antigen in association with MHC class 2 molecules. By processing and presenting antigen in different ways different antigen-presenting cells interact with different populations of lymphocytes. This is in part due to the way the antigen is handled and in part to the location of the particular antigen-presenting cell within the lymphoid system. The location of the main antigen-presenting cells of secondary lymphoid tissue (spleen and lymph node) is indicated below.

antigen-presenting cell		phago-cytosis	Fc/C3 receptors	class 2 MHC ex-pression	present to:
marginal zone macrophages	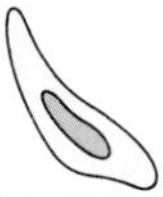	+	+	−	B
follicular dendritic cells	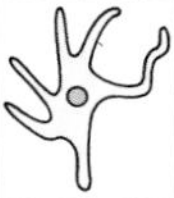	−	+	−	B
dendritic cells	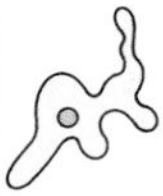	−	−	+	T
monocytes/ macrophages	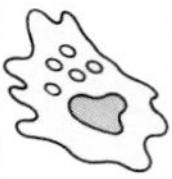	+	+	+/−	T + B
Langerhans cell	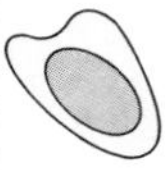	−	+	+	T

The second column header "characteristics" spans phago-cytosis, Fc/C3 receptors, class 2 MHC expression, and present to.

Fig.1.6 Chief characteristics of different antigen-presenting cells.

Marginal zone macrophages are present in the marginal zone of the splenic PALS and along the marginal sinus of lymph nodes. T independent antigens such as polysaccharides tend to localize on these cells, where they are often very persistent. Consequently they present antigens primarily to B cells.

Follicular dendritic cells are present in spleen and lymph node follicles where they appear to be tightly surrounded by lymphocytes. Complement fixing immune complexes localize on the surface of these cells via their Fc and C3 receptors, where they are presented mainly to B cells. This form of complex localization and presentation is apparently important in the development of B cell memory.

Antigen-presenting macrophages. Macrophages phago-cytose antigens, and some of them can also present it. The pools of phagocytosed antigen and surface antigen are distinct, and antigen is turned over fairly rapidly. Most of the recirculating macrophages of secondary lymphoid organs are seen in the medulla of the lymph nodes and the red pulp of the spleen whereas resident macrophages are particularly prevalent in the marginal zones.

Langerhans cells (veiled cells) are recirculating cells seen in skin which pick up antigen and transport it to the regional lymph nodes. They have a characteristic racket-shaped granule called the Birbeck granule (function unknown), and are rich in MHC class 2 molecules. In the lymph they are seen as veiled cells and in the lymph nodes as dendritic cells. U.V. irradiation of skin or treatment with skin sensitizing reagents induces emigration of the local Langerhans cells.

Dendritic (Interdigitating) cells, located in the T cell area of the lymph node carry MHC class 2 molecules and are highly active in presenting antigen to T helper cells. They are thought to be most important in the development of contact (delayed) hypersensitivity reactions.

Ia induction. A number of other cells including capillary endothelium and some endocrine cells, can present antigen in some circumstances. The cells develop MHC class 2 (Ia) molecules which confer the antigen-presenting function. Activated T cells, which release IFNγ actively induce Ia expression on some tissue cells.

Nurse cells are dendritic cells of the thymus, which are closely surrounded by lymphocytes. It has been suggested that they are important in the development of the T cell repertoire, but this is subject to debate.

PHAGOCYTES AND AUXILIARY CELLS

Reticuloendothelial system is the collective term for the long lived phagocytic cells distributed throughout the organs of the body. They are derived from bone marrow stem cells and most have been shown to have receptors for the Fc region of immunoglobulin and activated C3. Their function is to pick up antigenic particles and debris. Some of them have the ability to present antigen to lymphocytes. These cells include:

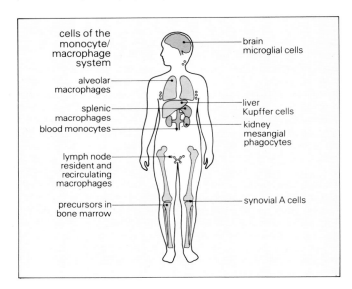

Fig.1.7 Phagocytes of the reticuloendothelial system.

Monocytes are circulating cells constituting about 5% of the total blood leucocytes. They have a well developed Golgi apparatus and many lysosomes. They migrate into the tissues, becoming macrophages.

Macrophages are large phagocytic cells found in most tissues and lining serous cavities and the lung. They are long-lived cells, and may remain in the tissues for years. Other macrophages recirculate through the secondary lymphoid organs, spleen and lymph nodes where they may function as APCs.

Kupffer cells are phagocytes which lie along the liver sinusoids. Much of the antigen entering the body through the gut is removed by these cells.

Mesangial phagocytes line the glomerular endothelium where the capillaries enter the Bowman's capsule.

Microglial cells are itinerant phagocytes of the brain.

Synovial A cells are one of the cell types which lie on the synovium, in contact with the synovial fluid, which lubricates the joint surfaces.

Granulocytes (polymorphs), recognizable by their multi-lobed nucleii and numerous cytoplasmic granules, constitute the majority of blood leucocytes. They are classified according to their histological staining as:

Neutrophils are professional phagocytes and the most abundant of the leucocytes (>70%). They spend less than 48 hours in the circulation before migrating into the tissues under the influence of chemotactic stimuli, where they phagocytose material and eventually die. They have receptors for Fc and activated C3 to facilitate uptake of opsonized particles.

Eosinophils comprise 2 - 5% of the blood leucocytes. Their granules contain a crystalloid core of a basic protein which can be released by exocytosis causing damage to a number of pathogens, particularly parasites. The granules also contain histaminase and aryl sulphatase which damp down inflammatory reactions.

Basophils constitute less than 0.5% of blood leucocytes. They mediate inflammatory reactions, and are in some ways functionally similar to mast cells.

Mast cells are present in most tissues, adjoining the blood vessels. They contain numerous granules with inflammatory mediators, which are released by triggering with C3a and C5a, or by crosslinking of surface IgE bound to their Fc$^\epsilon$ receptors. There are two types (connective tissue mast cells and mucosal mast cells) which differ in their response to drugs and stimuli, and in the blend of mediators they release.

Connective Tissue Mast cells (CTMC) are the main tissue fixed mast cell population. They are ubiquitous, contain large amounts of histamine and heparin, and unlike MMCs are susceptible to the action of sodium cromoglycate.

Mucosal Mast Cells (MMC) are either T cell derived or T cell dependent and are present in the gut and lung. They are increased in the gut during parasite infections and may recirculate.

LYMPHOID SYSTEM

Primary and Secondary lymphoid tissue. Lymphocytes are derived from the bone marrow stem cells. Immature cells develop in the primary lymphoid tissues - T cells in the thymus and B cells initially in the foetal liver and subsequently in the bone marrow. Mature cells seed the secondary lymphoid organs, the spleen, lymph nodes and collections of mucosal associated lymphoid tissues (MALT).

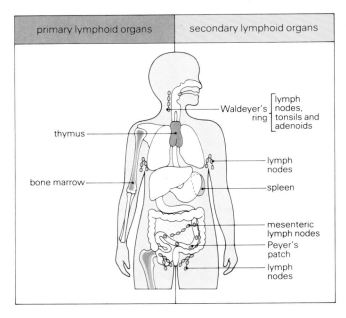

Fig.1.8 Major lymphoid organs and tissues.

Lymphocyte traffic / Recirculating cells. Lymphocytes leave the circulation by traversing specialized venules in the spleen, lymph nodes and MALT. These cell recirculate via the lymphatic system through chains of lymph nodes back to the circulation. Macrophages and Langerhans cells also recirculate from the periphery to the lymph nodes, bringing antigen into the nodes where they present it to lymphocytes.

High Endothelial Venules (HEV) are present in lymph nodes, spleen and the MALT. They are lined by distinctive columnar cells, and lymphocytes migrate from the circulation into the tissues at this point.

Right thoracic duct (TD) is the main lymphatic vessel through which recirculating cells pass, en route from the trunk internal organs and lower limbs, to the circulation. It drains into the left subclavian vein.

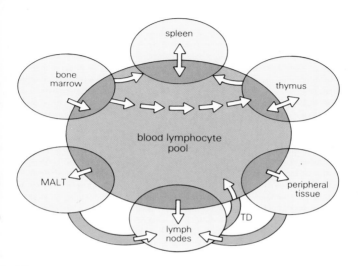

Fig.1.9 Lymphocyte traffic.

Lymphoid network is a system of vessels covering the entire body, which is responsible for draining the tissue, and returning the transudate to the blood. It also acts as a channel for the movement of antigens from the periphery to the lymph nodes, and for the recirculation of lymphocytes and macrophages.

Waldeyer's ring is the term for the lymphoid tissue of the neck and pharynx which includes the adenoids, tonsils and regional lymph nodes.

Lymph node shutdown. Under normal circumstances there is a steady efflux of lymphocytes from a lymph node, but when antigen enters the node of a sensitized animal, the emigration stops for a period of about 24 hours, referred to as shutdown.

Lymph nodes are encapsulated organs which punctuate the lymphoid network, and contain aggregations of lymphocytes and antigen presenting cells.

Afferent and Efferent lymphatics. Cells arrive in the lymph nodes via the HEV and afferent lymphatics which drain into the subcapsular sinus. From here they migrate across the node, or into specialized areas, and finally leave by the efferent lymphatic vessel.

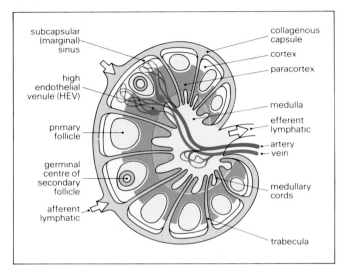

Fig. 1.10 The structure of a lymph node.

Lymph nodes are structurally organized into areas:
Cortex, the outer region contains mainly B cells. Lying within this region are follicles.

Lymphoid follicles are aggregations of closely packed lymphocytes and antigen-presenting cells. Unstimulated lymph nodes contain primary follicles, which develop into expanded secondary follicles after antigen stimulation.

Germinal centres are regions of rapidly proliferating cells seen in the centre of some secondary lymphoid follicles.

Paracortex contains mainly T cells, interspersed with inter-digitating cells rich in MHC class 2 antigens. These present antigens to the T cells.

Medulla contains relatively fewer lymphocytes, and more macrophages and plasma cells than other regions.

Medullary cords are strands of lymphocytes, both B and T cells, which extend into the medulla.

Spleen. This encapsulated secondary lymphoid organ, which lies in the peritoneum beneath the diaphragm and behind the stomach, contains two main types of tissue termed the red pulp and the white pulp.

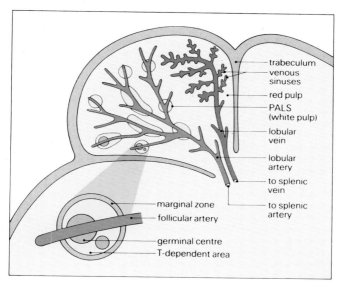

Fig.1.11 The structure of a spleen lobule.

Red pulp consists of a network of splenic cords and venous sinuses lined by macrophages, which effect the destruction of effete erythrocytes. Plasma cells may also be seen in this region of the spleen.

White pulp / PALS (Periarteriolar Lymphatic Sheath) contains the majority of the lymphoid tissue, distributed around the arterioles. T cells are mainly found around the central arteriole and B cells further out. The B cells may be organized into primary and secondary lymphoid follicles, with germinal centres. Phagocytes and antigen-presenting cells are also present in the follicles.

Marginal zone is the outer region of the PALS. It contains slowly recirculating B cells and marginal zone macrophages, which present T independent antigens to the B cells. Most lymphocytes enter the PALS via specialized capillaries in the marginal zone, and migrate out via bridging channels into the venous sinuses.

Thymus. This primary lymphoid organ overlies the heart. It is seeded by lymphoid stem cells from the bone marrow, which differentiate into T lymphocytes. The thymus is bilobed and is organized into lobules separated by connective tissue septae (trabeculae). Each lobule is divided into a cortex and a medulla.

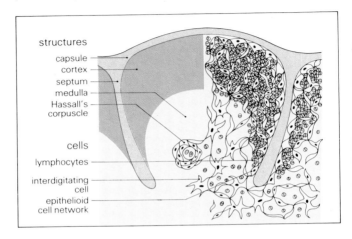

Fig. 1.12 The structure of a thymus lobule.

Thymocytes are thymic lymphocytes. The repertoire of T cell antigen receptors, and the capacity to distinguish self from non-self develop in the thymus, by interactions with antigen-presenting cells. There is considerable cell death, as well as proliferation.

Thymic cortex, the outer thymus zone, contains about 85% of the total thymocytes. These cells carry the T6 marker (humans), are relatively immature and divide rapidly.

Thymic medulla contains relatively few lymphocytes, but they are more mature than those in the cortex. Interdigitating antigen-presenting cells are also present; they carry MHC class 2 molecules are are thought to be important in the development of the thymocytes.

Thymic epithelial cells are a network of MHC class 2 molecule bearing epithelial cells which extend throughout the cortex and medulla.

Hassal's corpuscles are whorled structures possibly of epithelial cells seen in the medulla. Their function is unknown.

Mucosal Associated Lymphoid Tissue (MALT) is a general term for the unencapsulated lymphoid tissue, lymphocytes, antigen-presenting cells and plasma cells, which are seen in submucosal areas of the respiratory, gastrointestinal and urinogenitary systems. These protect potential sites of pathogen invasion.

Gut Associated Lymphoid Tissue (GALT) describes the MALT of the gut. The gut contains focal accumulations of lymphocytes in the lamina propria and Peyer's patches, both with a disproportionately large number of IgA producing B cells and plasma cells.

Peyer's patches are collections of lymphocytes in the wall of the small intestine which appear macroscopically as pale patches on the gut wall. The adjoining part of the intestinal mucosa lacks goblet cells and has a specialized epithelium which includes a unique cell - the membranous M cell. This region is permeable to antigens. Here also, IgA produced by local plasma cells is transported into the gut lumen. The Peyer's patches contain B and T cell areas and may have germinal centres. Lymphocytes enter the area via high endothelial venules.

Tonsil: a pharyngeal part of the MALT, particularly rich in B cells, arranged into follicles.

Secretory immune system refers to immune defences present in secretory organs, such as the salivary glands, mammary glands and MALT. The main protection is provided by secretory IgA (sIgA). Dimeric IgA is bound to a secretory piece on the basal surface of epithelial cells and transported across to the lumen. Although the newborn of some species are protected by maternal IgG which has crossed the placenta, in other species IgG secreted in the milk is the main form of protection. This is taken up from the gut of the neonate by a specialized transport system.

Bursa of Fabricius. This organ acts as a site of B cell development in birds. (Mammals do not possess this organ.) It develops as an outpushing of the endoderm near the end of the gut and becomes infiltrated with lymphocytic stem cells during embryonic development. It is a site of haemopoiesis as well as lymphopoiesis.

2 Antibodies and Antigens

ANTIBODY STRUCTURE

Antibodies are a class of serum proteins which are induced following contact with antigen. They bind specifically to the antigen which induced their formation.

Immunoglobulin (Ig) is a synonym for antibody. Most antibodies are weakly charged at neutral pH and are found in the gamma globulin fraction of serum.

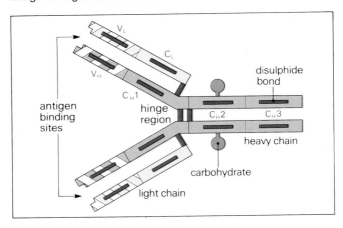

Fig.2.1 The basic structure of IgG.

Heavy chains and Light chains. Antibody molecules all have a basic four polypeptide chain structure consisting of two identical heavy (H) chains and two identical light (L) chains, stabilized and crosslinked by intrachain and interchain disulphide bonds (red). Heavy chains have carbohydrate (blue). Different antibody classes may consist of polymers of this four chain structure. Heavy chains are of five major types ($\gamma, \mu, \delta, \alpha, \epsilon$) depending on the antibody class, and consist of 450 - 600 amino acid residues. Light chains are of two major types (κ, λ) and have about 230 amino acid residues. Both heavy and light chains are folded into domains.

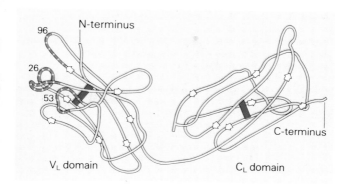

Fig.2.2 The basic folding pattern of the variable and constant domains of the light chain.

Domains are globular regions of protein. Antibody domains consist of 3 or 4 peptide loops stabilized by β-pleated sheet and an intrachain disulphide bond. Light chains have two domains and heavy chains have four or five.

The hinge region is a section of the heavy chain between the Fc and Fab regions which contains the inter-heavy chain disulphide bonds, and confers segmental flexibility on the antibody molecule.

Variable (V) and Constant (C) regions. Examination of the degree of amino acid variability between different antibody molecules of the same class shows that the largest amount of sequence variation is concentrated in the N-terminal domains of the light and heavy chains, hence this region is called the variable (V) region, while the remainder of the molecule, which has relatively little variation, is called the constant (C) region. The domains of antibody molecules are named according to whether they are in the variable or constant region of the molecule and according to whether they are on the light or heavy chain, eg V_H, C_H etc.

V_H & V_L are the variable domains of the heavy and light chains.

C_L & C_H1 are the constant domains of the light chain and the first constant domain of the heavy chain respectively.

$C\gamma$, $C\mu$, etc. Heavy chain domains are sometimes referred to by the class of antibody, for example, $C\mu1$ is the first constant domain of the μ heavy chain of IgM antibody.

ANTIBODY - STRUCTURAL VARIATIONS

Antibody molecules are structurally heterogeneous although they are all built up from units which have a basic four polypeptide chain structure.

Classes and subclasses. Antibodies may be grouped on the basis of structural similarities into different classes and subclasses depending on the nature of their heavy chains. Each class subserves different functions. In mammals there are five antibody classes - IgG, IgM, IgA, IgD and IgE. Some of these are further divided into subclasses. The number of subclasses in each class varies between different species, for example, in man there are four subclasses of IgG: IgG1 - IgG4.

Kappa & Lambda chains. Antibody light chains may also be divided into two types, namely κ and λ, depending on their constant domains. Both κ and λ chains can combine with any of the different heavy chain types.

The variability of antibodies is due to their being encoded by a number of genes, which are rearranged before they are expressed. Variation may be divided into three categories:

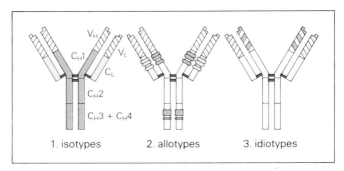

Fig. 2.3 Variability of immunoglobulin structure.

Isotypes. Variants which are present in all members of a species. Examples of isotypic variants are the different antibody classes and subclasses, where there are distinct gene loci for each variant.

Allotypes. Variants which are due to intraspecies genetic differences. Each individual has one particular allotype at each of its immunoglobulin gene loci, which often differ from those present in other individuals.

Idiotypes. Variants due to the large amount of structural heterogeneity in the immunoglobulin V regions. This is related to the production of a wide variety of different V regions to bind diverse antigens.

Kabat and Wu plot shows the amino acid sequence variability in immunoglobulins. Individual immunoglobulin molecules are sequenced and the number of different amino acids found at each position (A) and the frequency (B) of the most common is determined. Variability equals A/B.

Hypervariable regions and Framework segments. Using the Kabat and Wu technique on immunoglobulin V regions, it is found that the greatest variability is clustered in three hypervariable regions (red) which are separated by relatively invariant framework segments (yellow) as illustrated below for mouse V_H domains.

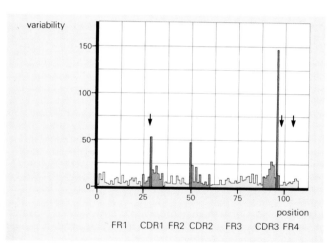

Fig.2.4 Kabat and Wu plot of light chain variability.

Complementarity Determining Region (CDR) is a part of the V region which forms the antigen binding site. A CDR is virtually synonymous with a hypervariable region.

Groups and Subgroups. The numerous V region domains can be classified into groups and subgroups according to similarities in the amino acid sequences of their frameworks. The genes encoding the proteins of a particular group lie adjacent in the V region DNA.

ANTIBODY FUNCTIONS

Antibodies are bifunctional molecules. Their first function is to bind to antigen and the second is to interact with host tissue. In this way, they act as an adaptor which can link the various antigens to the cells which effect immune reactions. The antigen binding site lies in the V region domains, while the C domains of the Fc region interact with cells of the immune system. Antibodies are synthesized in two different forms:

Membrane immunoglobulins are integral membrane proteins of B cells, acting as the B cells' antigen receptor.

Secreted immunoglobulins are structurally identical to their membrane counterparts except that they lack the trans-membrane section of amino acids at the C-terminus of membrane Ig. Secreted Igs are present in extracellular fluids and secretions.

Fc Receptors. These are integral membrane proteins which bind the Fc region of antibodies. They are class (and sometimes subclass) specific. Many antibody functions are effected by their binding to Fc receptors on cells.

IgG is the major serum immunoglobulin, and constitutes the majority of the secondary response to most antigens. It is transferred across the placenta (in humans) to provide protection in neonatal life. Most IgG subclasses bind C1q by sites in $C\gamma2$ to activate the classical complement pathway. IgG can act as an opsonin by cross-bridging antigen to Fc receptors on neutrophils and macrophages. It can also sensitize target cells for destruction by K cells.

IgM is a pentamer of the basic four chain structure. It is the first class to be produced both during the development of the immune system and during the primary response. It fixes complement very efficiently and may be the main component of the response to T-independent antigens.

IgA occurs as monomers, dimers and polymers of the basic four chain unit existing in man mostly as monomers, in other species as dimers. IgA is the most common immunoglobulin class in secretions, where it protects mucous membranes. It is also found in colostrum and is particularly important in protecting neonates of species which do not transfer IgG across the placenta.

J chain is a polypeptide present in polymeric Ig (IgM & IgA). It is manufactured by the B cell but is not encoded by the Ig genes.

23

Secretory component is a polypeptide synthesized by epithelial cells (rather than B cells) which becomes attached to secretory IgA dimers by disulphide bonds. The secretory component is an essential part of the IgA transport system, and it also protects the IgA from enzyme digestion within the gut.

IgD is a trace Ig in serum and acts as a cell surface receptor on many B cells. Its function is unknown. It may play a role in the control of B cell function and the development of memory, or may be simply an evolutionary relic.

IgE (reagin) binds to Fc receptors on mast cells and basophils where it sensitizes them to release pharmacological mediators after contact with antigen. IgE may be particularly important in protection against helminth infections, but it also mediates Type 1 hypersensitivity reactions.

Immunoglobulin	heavy chain	mean serum concentration (mg/ml)	sedimentation constant	molecular weight	molecular weight of heavy chain	number of heavy chain domains	carbohydrate (%)
IgG1	γ_1	9	7S	146,000	51,000	4	2-3
IgG2	γ_2	3	7S	146,000	51,000	4	2-3
IgG3	γ_3	1	7S	170,000	60,000	4	2-3
IgG4	γ_4	0.5	7S	146,000	51,000	4	2-3
IgM	μ	1.5	19S	970,000	65,000	5	12
IgA1	α_1	3.0	7S	160,000	56,000	4	7-11
IgA2	α_2	0.5	7S	160,000	52,000	4	7-11
sIgA	α_1 or α_2	0.05	11S	385,000	52-56,000	4	7-11
IgD	δ	0.03	7S	184,000	69,700	4	9-14
IgE	ε	0.00005	8S	188,000	72,500	5	12

Fig.2.5 Physicochemical properties of human immunoglobulin subclasses.

ANTIBODY GENES

Genome refers to the total genetic material in a cell. The genes for antibodies occur at three gene loci on separate chromosomes: these are κ, λ and heavy chain genes.

peptide	mouse	human
IgH	12	14
λ	16	22
κ	6	2

Fig.2.6 Chromosome locations of Ig genes.

Exons are gene segments which encode protein.

Introns are gene segments which lie between the exons. They do not encode protein but contain sequences important in gene control and the process of recombination.

Generation of diversity refers to the process by which the large number of antibody V regions are generated. This is acheived by 1) a large number of germ line V region genes in the separate gene pools for κ, λ and heavy chains, 2) recombination between V, D and J gene segments, 3) recombinational inaccuracies, 4) somatic point mutations, and 5) the varied combinations of light and heavy chains.

Germ line genes are passed down from one generation to the next. They may be altered during cellular development. The main modification of Ig genes is recombination between the V, J and D gene segments which encode the variable domain of heavy and light chains.

V genes encode the N-terminal 95 (approx.) amino acids of the V domains. The number of V genes at each locus varies between loci and species but may be up to several hundred.

J genes and D genes. To produce a gene encoding a heavy chain V region any one of the heavy chain V region genes is recombined with any one of a small number of D (diversity) and J (joining) genes to produce a VDJ gene. Recombination of light chains is similar except that they have no D gene segments and a V gene is recombined directly to a J gene. (J gene segments should not be confused with J chains.)

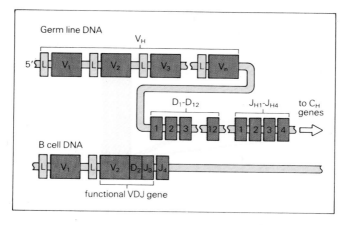

Fig.2.7 VDJ recombination.

Recombination is the process by which the gene segments are brought together and joined. This process depends on specific recombination sequences flanking each V, D and J gene segment. The recombination sequences appose these gene segments which are then enzymatically cut and rejoined to remove the intervening introns. A similar process, also called recombination, probably occurs in the chromosomal crossover during meiosis. The actual point at which recombination takes place may vary, as illustrated below for the recombination of the V_K21 and J_1 genes in three different myelomas. This gives rise to different base sequences encoding amino acids 95 and 96 thus providing an additional source of diversity.

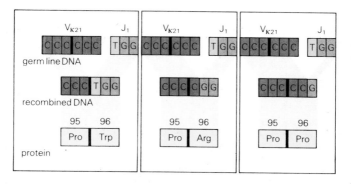

Fig.2.8 Light chain diversity created by variable recombination.

Somatic mutation is the process by which DNA base changes occur during the lifetime of a cell, producing point mutations in the encoded protein. There appears to be an active mechanism which inserts mutations into the gene region encoding the immunoglobulin V domains, which is activated during class switching. For this reason, IgG molecules usually differ from germ line encoded sequences, more than IgM molecules.

hnRNA, Primary transcript. The segment of gene containing the recombined VDJ (heavy chain) or VJ (light chain) region and the C region is transcribed into RNA. This still contains the gene sequences between the C and J regions and is called the primary transcript. These transcripts can be isolated from heteronuclear RNA (hnRNA), a population of large, heterogeneously-sized nuclear RNA molecules.

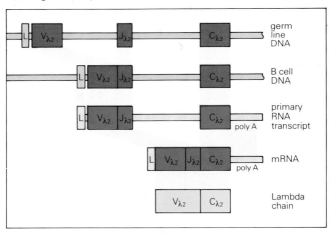

Fig.2.9 Lambda light chain production in the mouse.

Splicing. This is the process in which the primary hnRNA transcript is modified to remove the gene sequences between the J and C exons. The precise removal of the introns and rejoining to form mRNA depends on specific base sequences flanking the exons, called donor and acceptor junctions. The processed transcript is thus converted to mRNA which contains a poly-A-tail.

Leader (L). Each V gene is preceded by an exon encoding a leader polypeptide which is necessary for translation of the immunoglobulin across the membrane of the endoplasmic reticulum, but which is subsequently removed.

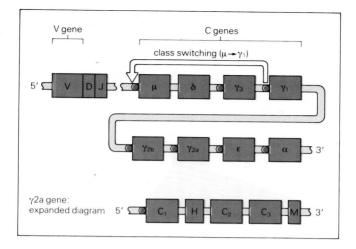

Fig.2.10 Constant region genes in the mouse.

C genes. The heavy chain constant region genes are arranged downstream (3') of the recombined VDJ gene. Each gene consists of a series of exons coding for the individual C domains, as well as separate exons for the hinge region and for the transmembrane segments of membrane immunoglobulins. The introns are removed during processing of the primary transcript. The primary transcript of the heavy chains can be processed in two different ways, to produce mRNA for either membrane or secreted immunoglobulin. To produce membrane immunoglobulin, the exons for the transmembrane segments are spliced to a point just within the final C domain, removing the translation stop signal at the end of that domain. If this does not occur the stop signal is retained and mRNA for secreted immunoglobulin is produced. Initially a B cell joins a μ gene to its VDJ gene, but other C genes may alternatively be linked to VDJ - this is called class switching.

Class Switching is a process by which the cell can switch the class of the immunoglobulin it produces while retaining the same antigen specificity. All the heavy chain constant region genes except δ are preceded by a switching sequence. The switch is probably effected by bringing a new gene up to the position occupied by the μ constant gene. The intervening C region genes are thought to be lost during this process. This is illustrated above for the switch from IgM to IgG1 production. The expression of δ genes, which lack a switch sequence, is controlled at the level of RNA processing.

ANTIBODY FRAGMENTS

Much of the early work on the elucidation of antibody structure was performed using fragments of antibodies prepared by a combination of methods including enzyme digestion and selective reduction of the interchain disulphide bonds. The fragments are separated chromatographically. Of particular interest are the Fab and F(ab')$_2$ fragments. Fab has one antigen combining site and so cannot crosslink antigenic determinants, while F(ab')$_2$ has two sites and can crosslink antigen. Both lack the Fc region, thus they are useful in determining which antibody effector functions are Fc dependent. The table below illustrates the structure of the fragments (yellow) and their means of production. IgG fragments are illustrated but analogous fragments can be made from other classes of immunoglobulins.

Fragment	Structure	Produced by
F(ab')$_2$	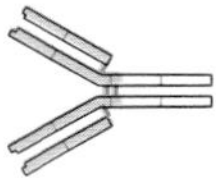	pepsin digestion
Fab'	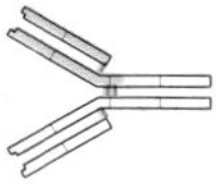	pepsin digestion and partial reduction
Fab	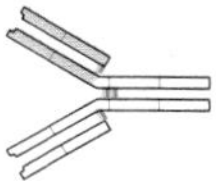	papain digestion
Fc	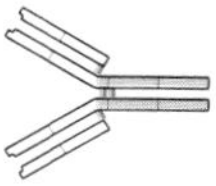	papain digestion
Facb	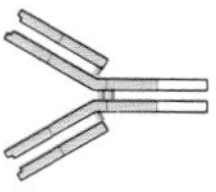	plasmin digestion
pFc'	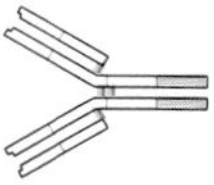	pepsin or plasmin digestion
Fd	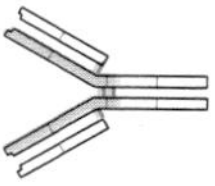	pepsin digestion partial reduction and reaggregation

Fig.2.11 Antibody fragments.

IDIOTYPES

Idiotypes are the particular determinants on antibody V regions and are identified by anti-idiotypic antibodies.

Cross-reactive Idiotypes (CRI) are analogous to cross-reacting antigens, in that they are idiotypes which occur on different Ig molecules. The immunoglobulin molecules may often be directed to the same antigen, or may have different binding specificities.

Recurrent and Dominant Idiotypes. It is sometimes observed that a particular idiotype is frequently seen in the immune response of different animals to a particular antigen. This is reffered to as a recurrent idiotype. If the idiotype constitutes a major proportion or the majority of the induced antibodies to the antigen, then it is a dominant idiotype.

Idi and Idx are abbreviations meaning a unique or individual idiotype (Idi) and a cross-reacting idiotype (Idx). These terms are applied in the context of particular antibody systems.

The majority of work on idiotypes has been performed on mice, using particular recurrent idiotypes. The ability to produce these idiotypes is usually determined by the presence of particular germ line V region gene sequences, such that the antibodies with that idiotype are produced either from the germ line genes, or from these genes with small numbers of mutations. The idiotypes are therefore usually associated with a particular immunoglobulin haplotype and are expressed strongly only in some strains.

Idiotype and/or Prototype Ab	Antigen	Strain	Ig Haplotype
TI5	PC	BALB/c	a
NP^b,B(1-8)	NP	C57BL/6	b
ABA(CRI)	ARS	A/J	e
A5A	Streptococcal carbohydrate	A/J	e
MOPC-460	TNP-Levan	BALB/c	a
Dex	α 1,3 Dextran	BALB/c	a
GAL	β 1,6 D-Galactan	BALB/c	a

Fig.2.12 Examples of mouse idiotypes.

ANTIGEN

Antigens are any molecules which are recognized by the immune system and induce an immune reaction.

Immunogen is an antigen which elicits a strong immune response, particularly in the context of protective immunity to pathogenic organisms.

Antigenic determinant is the part of the antigen to which an antibody binds. Antigens usually have many determinants which may be different from each other, or be repeated molecular structures.

Haptens and Carriers. Artificial antigens have been used to examine the immune response. In particular, small antigenic determinants (haptens) are covalently coupled to larger molecules (carriers). Haptens bind to antibodies but by themselves cannot elicit an antibody response. Haptens are usually recognized by B cells, and carriers by T cells.

Carrier Effect. This is the phenomenon where an optimal secondary antibody response is obtained when the hapten is coupled to the same carrier for both the primary and the secondary immunization. This is exemplified in Fig.2.14, 1 & 2 in the anti-DNP response following immunization with the carrier-hapten conjugates BSA-DNP and OA-DNP.

ARS	–	Azophenyl arsonate
BGG	–	Bovine gamma globulin
BSA	–	Bovine serum albumin
CGG	–	Chicken gamma globulin
DNP	–	Dinitrophenyl (hapten)
GAT	–	Glutamine Alanine Tyrosine copolymer
KLH	–	Keyhole Limpet Haemocyanin
NIP	–	4-hydroxy, 3-iodo, 5-nitrophenyl acetyl (hapten)
NP	–	4-hydroxy, 5-nitrophenyl acetyl (hapten)
OA	–	Ovalbumin
PC	–	Phosphorylcholine (hapten)
PLL	–	Poly-L-Lysine
(P,G)-A--L;	–	Synthetic polymers with an Ala-Lys (A–L)
(T,G)-A--L;		copolymer backbone substituted with a
(H,G)-A--L;		Glutamic acid (G) and either Phenylalanine (P)
		Tyrosine (T) or Histidine (H) side chains
PPD	–	Purified protein derivative (of tuberculin)
TNP	–	Trinitrophenyl (hapten)
TMA	–	Tetramethyl ammonium (hapten)

Fig.2.13 Commonly used carriers and haptens.

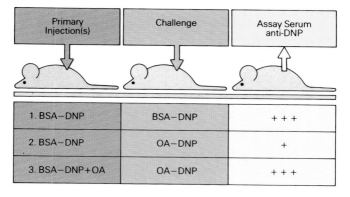

Primary Injection(s)	Challenge	Assay Serum anti-DNP
1. BSA–DNP	BSA–DNP	+ + +
2. BSA–DNP	OA–DNP	+
3. BSA–DNP+OA	OA–DNP	+ + +

Fig.2.14 Demonstration of the carrier effect.

Carrier Priming. The carrier effect may be bypassed by priming the animal to the new carrier (OA) before challenge (Fig. 2.14, 3).

T-dependent antigens need to be recognized by both T cells and B cells to elicit an antibody response. Most protein antigens fall into this category.

T-independent antigens are capable of stimulating B cells to produce antibody without T cell help. Most are large polymeric molecules with repeated antigenic determinants, which are only slowly degraded.

antigen	polymeric	polyclonal activation	resistance to degradation
lipopolysaccharide (LPS)	+	+ + +	+
Ficoll	+ + +	−	+ + +
dextran	+ +	+	+ +
levan	+ +	+	+ +
poly-D amino acids	+ + +	−	+ + +
polymeric bacterial flagellin	+ +	+ +	+

Fig.2.15 Commonly used T-independent antigens.

ANTIGEN/ANTIBODY INTERACTION

Antibodies bind specifically to the antigen which induces their formation. The antigen/antibody bond consists of multiple non-covalent interactions. These are reversible and so the Laws of Mass Action apply.

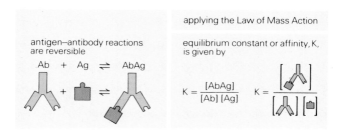

antigen–antibody reactions are reversible

applying the Law of Mass Action

$$Ab + Ag \rightleftharpoons AbAg$$

equilibrium constant or affinity, K, is given by

$$K = \frac{[AbAg]}{[Ab][Ag]}$$

Fig.2.16 Reversibility of the antigen-antibody bond and the calculation of antibody affinity.

Epitopes and Paratopes are part of a nomenclature used to describe the antigen/antibody interaction. An epitope is an antigenic determinant and the paratope, formed by the hypervariable loops of the V domains, is the part of the antibody which binds to the epitope.

Idiotopes are individual structural determinants on the antibody V region recognized by anti-idiotypic antibodies. They may be inside or outside the paratope.

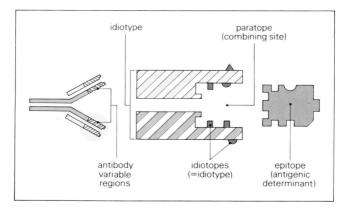

Fig.2.17 Nomenclature for the antibody V domains.

Antibody Affinity is a measure of the strength of the bond between a single antigen combining site and an antigenic determinant. It is dependent on a balance between the non-covalent interactions attracting the paratope and epitope and any repulsive forces generated by the overlap of adjoining electron clouds.

Antibody Valency is a measure of the number of binding sites on an Ig molecule. Each basic unit has two antigen combining sites so that dimeric IgA has four sites and IgM ten. The number of sites which are actually capable of binding to the antigen will also depend on the configuration of its determinants.

Antibody Avidity is a measure of the antigen/antibody binding strength, which depends on the affinity of the epitope/paratope reaction and the effective antibody valency. Since the strength of antibody/antigen binding is much enhanced when several bonds form, avidity is usually much greater than affinity.

Immune Complex. Antigen bound to antibody is termed an immune complex, but in the context of immunopathology complexes may also include complement components.

Cross-reaction. Some antisera are not totally specific for their inducing antigen but bind related (cross-reacting) antigens, either because the cross-reacting antigens share epitopes, or the epitopes are sufficiently similar in shape to bind the same antibody. For example, antiserum raised to antigen A, containing anti-X, anti-Y and anti-Z, can also bind to antigen B, either by shared epitope Y, or structurally similar epitope X'.

Polyfunctional binding sites are seen in some antibodies where more than one epitope can occupy the same paratope, though usually the two epitopes interfere, so that only one can occupy the combining site at one time.

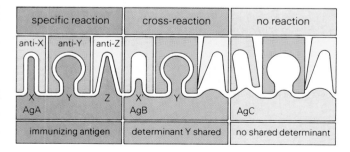

Fig.2.18 Specificity, cross-reactivity and non-reactivity.

3 The Immune Response

ADAPTIVE AND INNATE IMMUNITY

The immune response is mediated by a variety of soluble factors and cells, broadly divided according to whether they mediate adaptive (acquired) or innate (natural) immunity.

	Innate Immune System	Adaptive Immune System
	resistance not improved by repeated infection	resistance improved by repeated infection
soluble factors	lysozyme, complement, acute phase proteins eg. CRP, interferon	antibody
cells	phagocytes natural killer (NK) cells	T lymphocytes

Fig.3.1 The innate and adaptive immune systems.

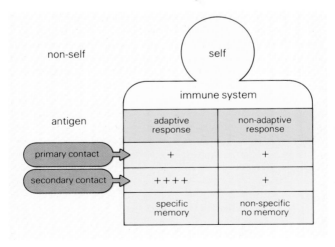

Fig.3.2 Primary and secondary immune responses.

35

Adaptive (Acquired) Immunity is specific for the inducing agent and is marked by an enhanced response on repeated encounters with that agent, thus displaying memory.

Innate (Natural) Immunity is dependent on a variety of effector mechanisms, which are neither specific for particular infectious agents nor improved by repeated encounters with the same agent.

Clonal Selection describes the way in which particular lymphocytes are activated. Each lymphocyte generates an antigen receptor with varying specificities (1,2,3 etc, Fig.3.3) so that when antigen encounters the immune system it binds specifically to only a few cells (2). These cells are stimulated to divide, so providing a large pool of effector cells and memory cells. Thus, antigen selects specific clones.

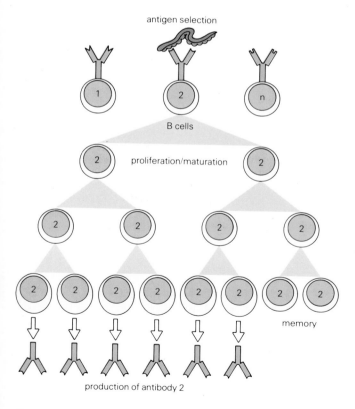

Fig.3.3 Clonal selection.

ANTIBODY RESPONSE

Following injection of an antigen, an antibody response develops which may be divided into four phases: a *lag phase* in which no antibody is detected, followed by a phase in which the antibody titres rise *log*arithmically, then *plateau* and *decline*, as the antibodies are catabolized, or cleared as complexes.

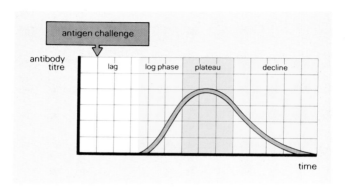

Fig.3.4 Graph showing the four phases of a primary antibody response.

Primary and Secondary antibody responses. The quality of the antibody response following the second (secondary) encounter with antigen varies from that following the first (primary) contact. The primary antibody response has a longer lag phase, reaches a lower plateau and declines more quickly than the secondary response. IgM is a major component of the primary response and is produced before IgG, whereas IgG is the main class represented in the secondary response. During their development some B cells switch from IgM production to IgG production and this is the basis of the change in antibody isotype seen in the secondary response. These differences between primary and secondary responses are most marked when the antigen stimulates both B cells and T cells (T dependent antigen).

Prime and Challenge are terms used to describe the administration of antigen either *in vivo* or to cells *in vitro*. The first administration is termed priming. This may be insufficient to engender a measurable response, but may still produce memory, or an enhanced secondary response. The term challenge is used loosely for any procedure which induces an immune response.

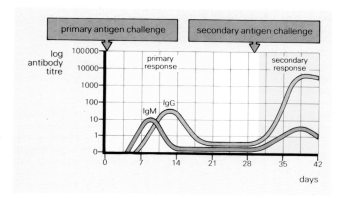

Fig.3.5 Primary and secondary antibody responses.

Affinity maturation describes the finding that the average affinity of the induced antibodies increases in the secondary response. This effect is largely confined to IgG and is most marked when a low antigen dose is given in the secondary injection. The low dose preferentially binds to high affinity B cell clones and activates them.

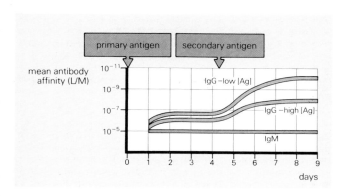

Fig.3.6 Affinity maturation.

Antiserum is serum from an animal containing specific antibodies, usually produced by repeated immunization.

Immunization is the procedure of antigen administration to induce antibodies or produce protective immunity.

CELL COOPERATION IN THE IMMUNE RESPONSE

Cell cooperation. Cooperation between the different types of cells involved in an immune response occurs at several levels. Phagocytes and antigen-presenting cells take up antigen in the periphery, process it and transport it to secondary lymphoid organs (spleen, lymph node, etc) where it is presented to lymphocytes in an immunogenic form. B cells produce antibody which binds to Fc receptors on phagocytes (as well as mast cells and K cells) so facilitating their uptake of antigen. T cells stimulated by antigen produce a variety of antigen specific and non-specific factors termed lymphokines, which help B cells to produce antibody and phagocytes to deal more effectively with pathogens.

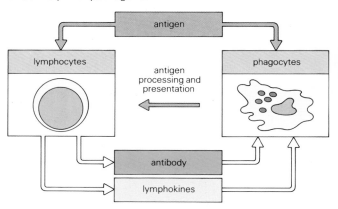

Fig.3.7 Interaction between lymphocytes and phagocytes.

Lymphokines are a group of molecules, other than antibodies, produced by lymphocytes which are involved in signalling between cells of the immune system. The group includes some interleukins, B cell growth and differentiation factors, interferon γ, and many less well characterized molecules, or 'activities'.

T cell help. To produce an antibody response to most antigens requires that both T cells and B cells recognize the antigen. Such antigens are called T dependent antigens to differentiate them from T independent antigens, which can stimulate B cells directly. T helper cells (TH) and B cells usually recognize different parts of the antigen, and the T cell delivers a signal to the B cell. This process is referred to as T cell help. The B cells

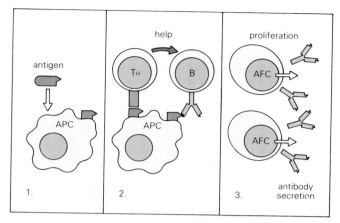

Fig.3.8 Overview of the immune response.

are stimulated to proliferate and differentiate into antibody forming cells (AFC) which secrete antibody. Antigen-specific help may be delivered by soluble factors or by direct cellular interaction. There is evidence that both mechanisms can occur, and in either case the cooperation may be genetically restricted. T cell help can also be signalled by non-specific factors which selectively stimulate cells close to the T cell.

Antigen processing. Antigen entering the immune system sometimes requires processing before it can be recognized by lymphocytes. Phagocytes which take up antigen can either degrade it completely in their phagolysosomes or can return partly degraded antigens to the cell surface where it is presented to the lymphocytes. The two pathways are apparently quite distinct. T cells appear to be able to recognize quite small antigen fragments, if appropriately presented, whereas B cells often only recognize larger, conformationally intact determinants.

Antigen presentation is the process by which antigen is presented to lymphocytes in a form they can recognize. This is a function of specialized antigen-presenting cells (APCs). For T helper cells and T cytotoxic cells to recognize antigen it must be presented in association with molecules encoded by the major histocompatibility complex (MHC). B cells and some T suppressor cells do not have this requirement. The form in which an antigen is presented determines whether it is immunogenic or tolerogenic, and affects the type of response made by lymphocytes.

ANTIGEN PRESENTATION

Antigens are recognized by T cells in association with MHC encoded molecules. This could occur in one of two ways as illustrated below for the presentation of antigen in association with an MHC Ia molecule to a T helper cell by a macrophage.

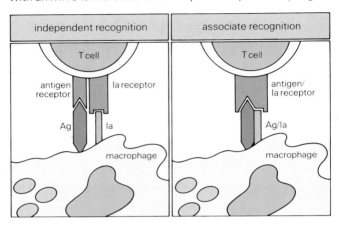

Fig.3.9 Antigen presentation by macrophages.

Independent recognition. This hypothesis proposes the existence of separate receptors on the T cell for antigen and the MHC molecule.

Associate recognition. In this hypothesis the processed antigen becomes physically associated with the MHC product and the combined unit is then recognized by a single receptor molecule.

Altered self. This is the idea that the MHC/antigen combination appears to the cell like an altered self-MHC molecule. This idea was developed to explain how T cell recognition of allogeneic cells and recognition of antigen could be effected by a single mechanism.

Class 1/Class 2 restriction. It is found that T cells recognize antigen in association with particular classes of MHC molecules. Generally speaking, cytotoxic T cells recognize antigen in association with MHC class 1 molecules (molecules which have one MHC-encoded chain associated with β_2-microglobulin) whereas helper T cells recognize antigen in association with class 2 molecules (molecules which have both chains encoded within the MHC, these have a more restricted tissue distribution than class 1 molecules).

A special nomenclature has been coined to describe the parts of the MHC molecule and how they associate with the antigen. These are illustrated below.

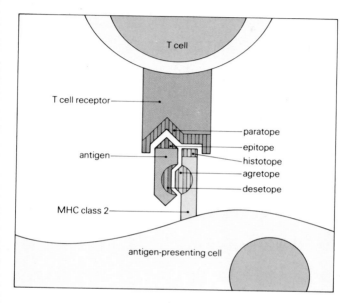

Fig.3.10 Antigen presentation - a hypothesis.

Agretope. This is the part of the MHC molecule which associates with the antigen (derivation: **a**nti**g**en **re**cognition).

Desetope. This is the part of the antigen which binds to the MHC molecule. It determines the orientation of the antigen and so which part will be presented to the T cell (derivation: **de**terminant **se**lection). Allotypically different class 2 molecules with different agretopes would vary in the way they associate with antigen, and thus in how they stimulate T cells. In this way they could determine immune response (Ir genes).

Histotope. This is the part of the MHC molecule which is recognized by the T cell.

The terms epitope and paratope are used in a way analogously to the terminology of antigen/antibody reactions.

MECHANISMS OF CELL COOPERATION

There is evidence for two mechanisms by which T cells help B cells. 1) T and B cells interact directly, linked by an antigen bridge and by recognition of MHC and processed antigen molecules expressed on the B cell. 2) T cells release helper factors which bind in association with antigen to antigen-presenting cells (APC). B cells recognize the factor and antigen.

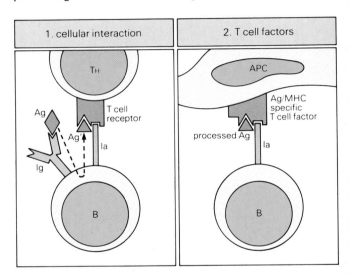

Fig.3.11 Two possible mechanisms of antigen-specific B cell activation by Tdep antigens.

Antigen bridge. This provides a way in which lymphocytes specific for a particular antigen can interact with each other. Each cell binds to separate epitopes on the same antigen molecule via their antigen receptors. This could occur in the interactions between T and B cells, and in the regulatory interactions involving T suppressor cells.

Helper/Suppressor factors released by T cells either enhance or suppress the response of other lymphocytes. They are often antigen specific. In some systems they act by binding to antigen-presenting cells and thus modify the responses of lymphocytes trafficking past. The classical helper factor is released by T$_H$ cells and acts on macrophages or B cells; it is thought to be MHC class 2 restricted. Suppressor factor is released by T$_S$ cells and acts primarily on T cells.

Genetically Restricted Factor (GRF) is released by macrophages, is class 2 restricted and induces TH cells. It has been observed to act in an antigen-specific manner in some experiments.

Interleukins. These are a group of antigen non-specific factors involved in lymphocyte activation and differentiation.

Interleukin 1 (IL-1)/Lymphocyte Activating Factor (LAF), is produced by macrophages and other antigen-producing cells. It acts on T cells to induce IL-2 receptors.

Interleukin 2 (IL-2)/T Cell Growth Factor (TCGF) is produced by activated T cells. It is necessary for the long term proliferation of T cells and can also act on previously stimulated B cells.

Interleukin 3 (IL-3) is one of the colony stimulating factors (CSF), produced by cell lines of several lineages which induces proliferation of lymphocytes.

B cell Stimulating Factors (BSF). This is the term for factors which act on B cells, including:

B Cell Growth Factor (BCGF). Two separate molecules which induce activated B cells to proliferate.

T Cell Replacing Factor (TRF)/B Cell Differentiation Factor (BCDF). A group of molecules which are required for B cell differentiation. Some preparations contain BCGF.

	source	target	effect
Interleukin 1 (LAF)	macrophage and other cells	T and B cells	promotes multiplication and activation
Interleukin 2 (TCGF)	Ly1$^+$, 23$^-$ T cell in presence of macrophage	T cells	proliferation of activated T cells
T cell replacing factor (TRF)	Ly1$^+$, 23$^-$ T cell in presence of macrophage	B cells	B cell differentiation
B cell growth factor (BCGF)	Ly1$^+$, 23$^-$ T cell in presence of macrophage	B cells	synergizes with IL-1 in B cell activation

Fig.3.12 Antigen non-specific factors.

SOLUBLE MEDIATORS OF IMMUNITY

Signalling between leucocytes is effected by a variety of soluble factors. These factors were originally identified in lymphocyte tissue culture supernatants. The supernatants often contained a large number of different factors and their activity was measured in biological assays so it was not clear whether one molecule could have several different effects or if several molecules were equally effective in any particular assay. The term 'lymphokines' was coined to describe such lymphocyte-derived factors, which were classed according to their activity. With improved biochemical techniques, some of these factors have been fully characterized and are now more rigorously classified as interleukins, interferons, helper and suppressor factors and so on. Other lymphocyte and macrophage derived factors are listed below.

Migration Inhibition Factor (MIF). MIF is a molecule produced by antigen-stimulated T cells, which inhibits the migration of macrophages. It is important in causing macrophage accumulation in cell-mediated immune reactions.

Leucocyte Migration Inhibition Factor (LIF) has a similar action to MIF but with wider cell specificity.

Macrophage Activation Factor (MAF) increases microbicidal and cytotoxic capacity of macrophages; this is now known to be partly due to interferon γ (IFNγ).

Eosinophil and Neutrophil Chemotactic Factors (ECF & NCF) attract these cells to sites of inflammation.

Colony Stimulating Factors (CSF) are molecules which induce proliferation of particular cell populations. Different CSFs act on different cell types.

Macrophage Fusion Factor (MFF) is thought to be involved in the cell fusion which produces giant cells.

Transfer Factor is a group of low molecular weight antigen specific factors which can transfer cutaneous delayed hypersensitivity. They are extracted from leucocytes.

Soluble Immune Response Suppressor (SIRS) produced by suppressor T cells inhibits antibody (plaque) forming cells *in vitro*. It acts primarily through macrophages.

Tumour Necrosis Factor (TNF) produced by macrophages is cytotoxic for some tumour cells and some parasites.

IMMUNOSUPPRESSION

Immunosuppression describes the measures which are used to reduce the immune response, particularly in transplantation surgery, to prevent graft rejection and in the control of autoimmune disease. Most measures are not antigen specific although some of the drugs used have a greater effect on the immune system than on other tissues.

Steroids, including glucocorticosteroids and corticosteroids have a wide acting immunosuppressive effect. Macrophages are particularly sensitive, and steroids inhibit their activation and secretion of neutral proteases, thereby reducing inflammation. Steroids inhibit the release of arachidonic acid which is the substrate for the lipoxygenase and cyclo-oxygenase pathways which form various inflammatory mediators, including prostaglandins and leukotrienes. Steroids strongly inhibit the primary antibody response and reduce the numbers of circulating T cells, particularly T helper cells.

Azathioprine and 6-mercaptopurine. Metabolites of these drugs depress cellular activity. Monocytes are reduced and K cell activity is greatly inhibited.

Cyclophosphamide and Chlorambucil are alkylating agents which damage DNA and prevent is replication. They act primarily on lymphocytes and strongly inhibit antibody responses, but have little effect on phagocyte activity. Experimentally, cyclophosphamide prevents B cells regenerating their surface immunogobulin. It has also been used to potentiate tolerization.

Cyclosporin-A is a fungal metabolite which interferes with early events in lymphocyte activation and transformation. It does not, however, affect lymphoblasts nor is it anti-mitotic or cytotoxic. It primarily affects T cells (also B cells in man), and is becoming the drug of first choice in transplantation surgery. Complications of cyclosporin therapy are usually caused by its nephrotoxicity.

Anti-lymphocyte globulin is an antibody raised to lymphocytes. Experimentally it inhibits T cell function and has also been used in human grafting.

Irradiation, by X rays given either locally or generally has an immunosuppressive effect. T helpers and antigen-presenting cells are more affected than T suppressors although very high doses will effectively eliminate all lymphocytes, including stem cells.

IMMUNOREGULATION

The immune response is regulated by lymphocytes through positive and negative controls, as well as feedback from soluble factors including antigen, antibody, lymphokines and interleukins.

Antibody feedback. Antibody regulates its own level of synthesis in several ways. The following are important: (1) binding to antigen and thus preventing the antigen from activating lymphocytes: (2) binding to Fc receptors on B (and possibly Tγ) cells. In the presence of antigen this causes crosslinking of the antigen receptors and Fc receptors which is inhibitory to the cells: (3) antibody/antigen complement fixing complexes localize in germinal centres where they stimulate B and T cells and induce memory.

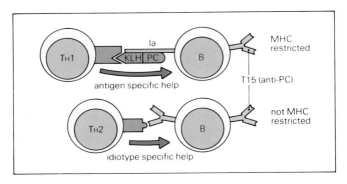

Fig.3.13 Antigen specific and idiotype specific Tн cells.

Immune regulation falls into three classes:
Antigen specific interactions are confined to cells which bind a particular antigen. These are mediated either by antigen specific factors or by direct cell/cell contact across an antigen bridge. The interaction is usually MHC restricted.

Idiotype specific interactions are confined to cells and antibodies expressing particular idiotypes on their antigen receptors; not usually MHC restricted. These two types of interaction are illustrated above for the antigen (KLH) acting as carrier, interacting with a B cell producing the T15 idiotype antibody to the hapten phosphorylcholine (PC).

Non-specific interactions affect lymphocytes regardless of their idiotype or antigen specificity. In practice the structural organization of the lymphoid system means that non-specific signals are localized in their effects.

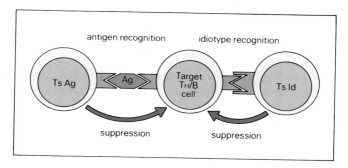

Fig.3.14 Antigen specific and idiotype specific T-suppressor cells.

Suppression. A regulatory group of T cells (T suppressors) are responsible for controlling the activity of T helper and B cells. Suppression is antigen-, idiotype- or non-specific. Antigen-specific suppression is often MHC restricted. The evidence points to the requirement for the T suppressor cell and the target cell to share I-J regions, in the mouse. Since the I-J region does not encode a separate protein, but lies within the region encoding class 2 (Ia) molecules, it is uncertain how the region could control suppressive interactions. Possibly the interactions involve Ia molecules which have become modified by gene products from loci outside the MHC. Suppression mediated by T cells is one mechanism by which the immune system could prevent the development of immune reactions to self molecules. Suppression is an active process and can be differentiated from tolerance by transferring the suppression with T cells.

Contrasuppression. This is the action of a group of T cells which act on T helper cells to render them resistant to suppression. Their significance is still debated.

TH1, TS1 etc are functional types of T-helper and T-suppressor cells. Ts1 and TH1 are antigen specific, Ts2 and TH2 are idiotype specific and Ts3 is non-specific.

Suppressor macrophages. This is a functional description of the action of macrophages in some experimental systems. The suppression is non-specific and is often mediated by prostaglandins.

IMMUNE RESPONSE GENES

Responder and Non-responder. Inbred strains of animals produce a characteristic level of immune response to injected antigens. Strains which produce high levels are responder, others are low responder or non-responders. The status depends mainly on MHC-linked immune response genes, and varies for different antigens.

Immune Response (Ir) genes. A large number of gene loci determine the level of immune response to an antigen. Ir genes act on antigen processing and presentation, cell cooperation, the repertoire of antigen receptors and the way T cell populations are activated. The most important Ir genes have been mapped to the MHC, particularly to the loci encoding class 2 MHC molecules.

Complementation. Ir genes are dominant and F_1 animals of low x high responders are high responders, but in some instances a low x low responder cross also produces a high responder; this is termed complementation. The term also applies to other gene systems.

Repertoire is the sum total of antigen receptors produced by the immune system. The B and T cell repertoires of an individual differ in the way they recognize antigen.

Holes (in the repertoire) are a way of explaining the non-responder status of an animal by saying that it lacks some particular antigen receptor.

Biozzi mice are strains genetically inbred to give high or low antibody responses to an antigen (originally sheep red blood cells). At least 10 separate Ir gene loci control responsiveness

macrophage function	low responder	high responder
1. antigen uptake	+++	+
2. lysosomal enzyme activity	+++	+
3. intracellular degradation of antigen	+++	+
4. surface persistence of antigen	+	+++

Fig.3.15 Macrophage functions in high and low responder mice.

in these animals. The high and low responder strains differ in the way their macrophages handle antigens (see Fig.3.15).

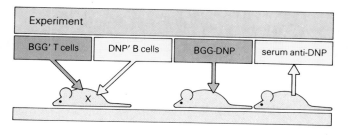

experiment	T cells	B cells	recipient	response
1	C	C	CxD	+
2	D	D	CxD	+
3	C	D	CxD	−
4	D	C	CxD	−
5	CxD	D	CxD	+

Fig.3.16 Genetic restriction in T/B cooperation.

Genetic restriction describes the finding that cells cooperate most effectively when they come from the same strain. The requirement is generally that the cells should share the same MHC haplotype. Genetic restriction is seen in macrophage/T cell interactions and in T/B cooperation. The effect occurs both in responses which require direct cell/cell contact and in some interactions mediated by soluble factors. This is illustrated above in an experiment where irradiated (X) animals of MHC type CxD were reconstituted with T cells primed to carrier (BGG') and B cells primed to hapten (DNP'). After challenge with BGG-DNP the response to DNP was measured. A response is obtained where T and B cells share at least one haplotype (C or D).

Clonal restriction. This refers to an immune response produced by a limited number of clones, an example of which is seen in the production of dominant idiotypes to some antigens in particular mouse strains.

IDIOTYPE NETWORKS

Anti-idiotypes (anti-Id). These are antibodies which react with the antigenic determinants (idiotopes) on the V region of other antibodies. Since anti-idiotypes can bind to T and B cells' antigen receptors they are often as efficient as antigen in stimulating these cells.

Jerne's Network hypothesis. This theory, as originally formulated, stated that since the repertoire of shapes that antibodies can bind to is virtually unlimited, and since antibodies themselves have an enormous variety of idiotypic shapes, they may interact with each other specifically to form an idiotypic network.

Network Theory is an extension of Jerne's hypothesis proposing that lymphocytes as well as antibodies can modulate the activity of others via their receptors.

Ab1, Ab2 etc. This is a nomenclature used when describing idiotype networks, where Ab1 is antibody directed towards an external antigen and carries a particular set of idiotypes. Ab2 is a population of antibodies directed towards idiotypes on Ab1. Ab3 is directed towards idiotypes on Ab2 and so on.

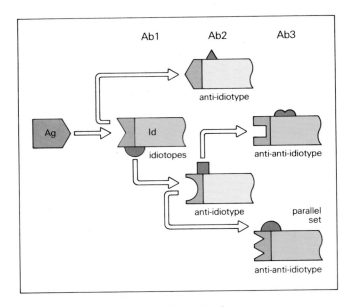

Fig.3.17 Jerne's Network hypothesis.

Branching describes the degree of heterogeneity in a network of idiotypic reactions. For example, if Ab2 recognizes a large number of different idiotopes on Ab1, the network is said to be highly branched.

Site associated and Site non-associated idiotopes. Idiotopes associated with the antigen combining site can be distinguished from idiotopes outside the combining site because anti-idiotypic antibody recognizing site associated idiotopes can be inhibited from binding to the idiotype by antigen (hapten) whereas anti-idiotype to non-site idiotopes is not inhibited.

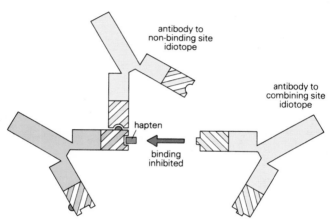

Fig.3.18 Distinction between idiotopes inside and outside the antibody combining site.

Internal image anti-idiotype. If a site associated anti-idiotype binds to the paratope of the idiotype in the same way that the antigen does, then the antigen and the anti-idiotype may have the same shape. In this case the anti-idiotype is said to be an internal image of the antigen - internal because it is generated by the immune system itself as opposed to the foreign antigen which is external.

Parallel Sets are antibody molecules which share an idiotope but are directed towards different antigens. According to the network theory they may be regulated concomittantly.

The diagram opposite illustrates a network consisting of antigen and a series of receptors, which may be on antibodies (Ab1, Ab2 etc.) or could be idiotypes on T cells.

TOLERANCE

Tolerance is the acquisition of non-responsiveness to a molecule recognized by the immune system. Whether a molecule induces an immune response or tolerance is largely determined by the way in which it is first presented to the immune system.

Tolerogen is a molecule which induces tolerance.

Tolerize means to administer a molecule in a way which makes an animal or cell population tolerant to it.

Either B cells or T cells (or both) can become tolerant to a molecule, and since an antibody response to most antigens requires T/B cooperation, tolerance in either cell population will produce overall tolerance. Conversely, if only B cells are tolerant the T cells may still be able to produce a cell-mediated immune response.

B cell tolerance. Generally speaking immature cells are more susceptible to tolerance than mature cells and can be tolerized by smaller doses of tolerogen. The dose of antigen and the way it is presented are critical. Ways or producing B cell tolerance are shown below.

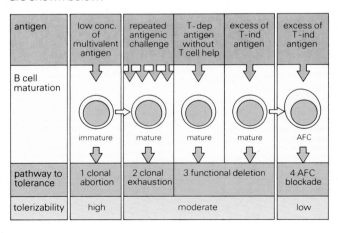

antigen	low conc. of multivalent antigen	repeated antigenic challenge	T-dep antigen without T cell help	excess of T-ind antigen	excess of T-ind antigen
B cell maturation	immature	mature	mature	mature	AFC
pathway to tolerance	1 clonal abortion	2 clonal exhaustion	3 functional deletion		4 AFC blockade
tolerizability	high	moderate			low

Fig.3.19 Pathways to B cell tolerance.

Clonal deletion: tolerance induced by the specific elimination of clones of antigen-reactive cells. Where reactive B cells are present, but unable to respond due to lack of T cell help, this is a functional deletion. Since potentially reactive B cells are often found in tolerant animals, this idea has become modified to the concept of clonal abortion.

Clonal abortion is similar to clonal deletion, except that the antigen reactive cells are not eliminated, they are still present, but are rendered inactive.

Clonal exhaustion: tolerance caused by repeated antigen stimulation, where antigen-reactive cells are activated so that the pool of mature cells becomes exhausted.

Antibody Forming Cell (AFC) blockade. Very large amounts of T independent antigens may interfere with antibody secretion. It is difficult to tolerize AFCs.

T cell tolerance. T cells are more easily tolerized than B cells. Once established, the duration of T cell tolerance in an animal is usually longer than that of the B cell tolerance. Immature T cells may be clonally aborted. Mature T cell populations can be functionally deleted depending on how antigen is presented to them, and they are also susceptible to the action of T suppressors.

High zone and Low zone tolerance. Tolerance is best induced by high antigen doses (high zone) which tolerize B cells. However, some antigens in minute doses (low zone) - much less than would be immunogenic - can also tolerize an animal by inducing T suppressor cells.

Neonatal tolerance. Neonatal animals are very susceptible to the induction of tolerance, due to the general immaturity of their immune systems. Consequently, tolerance induced at this stage of life is very persistent.

Self tolerance. It is observed that animals generally tolerate all their own tissues. If they do not, autoimmune disease may result. Self tolerance is thought to be due to clonal abortion of cells in the neonatal period: as new mature lymphocytes develop they too are aborted just when they are most susceptible to tolerization. This system is backed up by suppressor T cells.

Enhancement includes ways of inducing tolerance in transplantation surgery, where the graft survival is enhanced. The mechanism often involves interference with antigen presentation, for example by the administration of anti-Ia antibody to block T cell recognition of antigen in association with Ia (MHC class 2) molecules.

IMMUNOPOTENTIATION

Biological Response Modifiers (BRM) are compounds which modify an immune response, usually enhancing it. This includes immunopotentiating bacterial products, chemicals such as polynucleotides, physiologically active molecules such as thymic hormones and interferon, as well as the true adjuvants which are administered with the antigen. A number of these substances have been used in an attempt to potentiate immune reactions in cancer patients and people who suffer from immunodeficiency. Bacterial products include:

BCG (Bacillus Calmette Guerin) a live non-virulent strain of *Mycobacterium bovis*. It is used in vaccines for immunization against tuberculosis.

Muramyl Dipeptide (MDP) is the smallest adjuvant active part of BCG extractable from the cell wall.

Corynebacterium parvum induces lymphoid hyperplasia and activates macrophages.

Bordetella pertussis produces a lymphocytosis promoting factor (LPF) which is a T cell mitogen and an immunostimulant. *B. pertussis* causes whooping cough.

Adjuvants. These are compounds which enhance the immune response when administered with antigen producing higher antibody titres and prolonged production. The distinction between primary and secondary immune responses becomes blurred when adjuvants are used. Commonly used adjuvants include:

Incomplete Freund's Adjuvant (IFA) is a stable water in oil emulsion which forms an antigen depot.

Complete Freund's Adjuvant (CFA) is consituted as above but with the addition of killed *M. tuberculosis*.

Alum where the antigen is coprecipitated in alum.

Thymic hormones are factors produced by the thymus which play a role in the differentiation and development of T lymphocytes within the thymus and in their maintenance in the periphery. Some of these factors have been isolated from thymic epithelium, and they tend to decline with age concomitantly with thymic atrophy. (* = those which have been made artificially.)

name	chemistry	comment
Thymosin (fraction 5)*	α, β and γ polypeptides α-1-sequenced 28 amino acids MW – 3,108	some produced in thymic epithelial cells
Thymopoietin 1 and 2	sequenced; 49 amino acids MW – 5,562	produced only in thymus, activity in pentapeptide (TP-5)*
Thymic humoral factor (THF)	31 amino acids MW 3,220	partially sequenced
Thymostimulin (TP-1)	group of peptides	least well characterized
Thymulin Facteur thymique serique (FTS)*	9 amino acids	present in serum, disappears after thymectomy

Fig.3.20 Thymic hormones and factors.

4 Histocompatibility Loci and Transplantation

MHC GENES AND PROTEINS

Major Histocompatibility Complex/System (MHC/MHS) is a cluster of genes important in immune recognition and signalling between cells of the immune system. The gene complex was originally identified as a locus encoding molecules present on cell surfaces, such that animals which differed at this locus would rapidly reject each others tissue grafts. All mammals have an MHC:

H-2 is the mouse MHC and
HLA is the human MHC.

MHC antigens/specificities. The MHC encodes a large number of different proteins, and since many of them are polymorphic they are recognized as *antigens* when transferred between strains and can be identified by specific allo-antisera. In some cases, MHC molecules are identified by the reactions which they induce in cells of a different strain - in this case the molecule(s) inducing the reactions are termed MHC specificities. MHC antigens may be classified according to their overall structures into 3 groups.

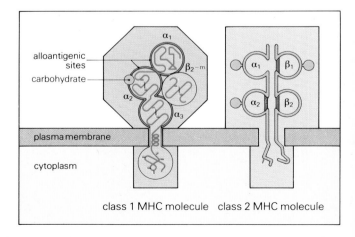

Fig.4.1 Class 1 and class 2 MHC molecules.

Class 1 MHC molecules are integral membrane proteins found on the surface of all nucleated cells and platelets. They are the classical transplantation antigens involved in graft rejection. Class 1 molecules have one polypeptide chain encoded by the MHC, which traverses the plasma membrane. The extracellular portion is folded into three globular domains (designated α_1, α_2 and α_3) which are non-covalently associated with another peptide - β_2-microglobulin. The polymorphism of class 1 molecules is confined to the MHC-encoded peptide. Class 1 MHC molecules are recognized by cytotoxic T cells, which can distinguish allogeneic sites in the α_1 and α_2 globular domains.

β_2-microglobulin is a polypeptide chain encoded by genes outside the MHC. It has a single domain which has structural homologies with Ig (and MHC) domains. It is necessary for transport of the MHC molecule to the cell surface and for its expression by the cell.

Domains (MHC) are globular regions of protein stabilized by secondary interactions and sometimes by disulphide bonds. The domains of MHC proteins are structurally related to each other, to the domains in Ig molecules and to the T cell surface molecule Thy.

Class 2 MHC molecules are expressed on B cells, macrophages, monocytes, various antigen-presenting cells and some T cells. They consist of two non-covalently linked peptides (α and β), both encoded by the MHC, which traverse the plasma membrane, each having two domains on the outside of the cell. Both chains can be polymorphic, although there is more structural variation in the β chains. Class 2 molecules are required to present antigen to T cells, in T/B cooperation to produce antibody, and in regulatory interactions between T cells. For this reason they affect immune responsiveness and the genes which encode them were initially identified as immune response genes.

Ia antigens. These molecules were originally identified as class 2 proteins encoded by the mouse MHC I-A subregion, but this term is now often more loosely used as a generic term for any class 2 MHC molecule.

Class 3 MHC molecules. Several complement components are encoded within the MHC, including B, C2 and C4, both in man and mouse. They are termed class 3 molecules. The reason for their location in this gene complex is uncertain, and could be a coincidental consequence of lying between sets of closely linked class 1 and class 2 genes.

GENETICS OF THE MHC

The MHC contains many separate genes and in man, for example, they occupy about 1/3000th of the total genome. It is remarkable, firstly, in that the MHC class 1 and class 2 molecules have an enormous amount of structural poly-morphism, and secondly, the rate of gene alteration within this locus is the highest yet observed.

Polymorphism refers to the large number of variants seen in different individuals at the same gene locus and hence in the proteins which that locus encodes. The variation is not scattered randomly throughout the molecules but tends to be concentrated in particular areas, especially in those sites which are recognized by cells of different strains, that is in allogeneic reactions.

Gene conversion is a process by which related genes exchange genetic information. This process is thought to occur between class 1 MHC genes and genes of the Qa locus, and so may contribute to MHC polymorphism.

MHC genes are expressed codominantly, for example, antisera to the $H-2^b$ and $H-2^k$ haplotypes (anti-b and anti-k) kill

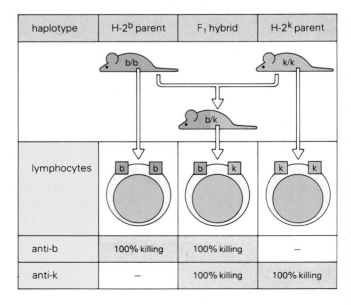

Fig.4.2 Codominant expression of MHC antigens.

cells of the haplotype to which they were raised and both kill cells of the F_1 hybrid, thus indicating that the F_1 cells express both parental haplotypes.

Terms used to describe MHC genetics include:

Genotype is the genetic composition of an animal.

Phenotype is the observed characteristics, which depends both on the genotype and how the genes are expressed.

Haplotype is a set of genes located on a single chromosome, and the characteristics dependent on them. In normal populations the maternal and paternal chromosomes differ, so an individual has two haplotypes of each set of genes. Inbred strains of animals have been produced so that each autosome pair is homozygous.

Inbred strains are produced by repeated brother x sister mating in successive generations, giving a strain with identical sets of autosomes. If by chance, a pair of identical chromosomes occurs in the F_1 of a brother x sister mating, inbreeding ensures that that pair remains fixed in the genome of subsequent generations. By repeated inbreeding, all the chromosome pairs become (and will remain) homozygous.

Recombinant strains are produced by crossing different inbred strains. On rare occasions, crossing over occurs in the F_1 animal so that the affected chromosome has different haplotypes at each end. Recombinant strains are used to identify the segment of chromosome responsible for particular characteristics.

Recombinant inbred strains are produced by crossing strains (a x b) and then inbreeding the offspring. This gives strains which have identical sets of chromosomes but each set will be either of the a type or the b type at random. These animals are used to determine which chromosomes carry the genes for each characteristic.

Congenic strains are bred to be identical to each other except at some chosen gene locus.

Linkage occurs between nearby genes on the same chromosome so that they tend to be inherited together.

Linkage disequilibrium refers to the finding that some pairs of genes are found together more frequently than would be expected by chance, that is, more often than the product of their individual gene frequencies.

H-2 – THE MOUSE MHC

The H-2 region lies on chromosome 17 and is divided into four main regions - K, I, S and D.

H-2K and H-2D encode class 1 molecules, the classical transplantation antigens (and class 1 pseudogenes).

Pseudogenes have sequence similarities to normal genes but they lack segments required for their expression.

H-2I encodes class 2 molecules. Originally, genetic mapping divided the region into 5 loci - IA, IB, IC, IJ and IE, but analysis of the DNA sequence shows that it encodes only two class 2 proteins, the α and β chains of Ia and Ie. The α chain of Ie is encoded in IE and the other chains in IA. Consequently, IB has been amalgamated into IA, and IC into IE. The IJ region does not encode a peptide directly, but may control Ts cell activity.

H-2S contains genes for the class 3 (complement) components C2, B, C4(Ss) and Slp.

Slp (sex-limited protein) is a non-functional variant of C4.

H-2G, a locus (not illustrated) between H-2S and H-2D, encodes enzymes unrelated to immune functions.

Qa and Tla loci contain genes for more than twenty-five class 1 molecules, but only those shown have been unequivocally detected on T cells. They may function in haemopoietic differentiation, act as target molecules for NK cells or be a source of DNA for gene conversion with class 1 molecules.

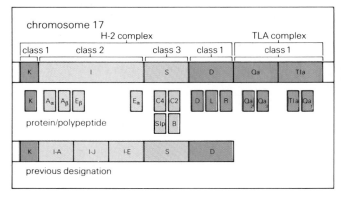

Fig.4.3 The mouse MHC.

HLA – THE HUMAN MHC

The HLA (Human Leucocyte Antigen) region lies on chromosome 6 and is divided into 4 main regions, A, B, C and D. Although the functions of the human MHC are less well studied than those of the mouse, evidence implies that class 1 and 2 moleucles have similar functions in each species.

HLA-A, -B and -C loci encode class 1 MHC molecules. The A and B loci show the greatest polymorphism with 23 and 49 haplotypes respectively. Only 8 haplotypes have been defined for the C locus so far.

HLA-D loci encode class 2 MHC molecules. Three gene loci have been identified, SB, DC and DR although the precise gene order is not determined. (A new nomenclature DP, DQ and DR has been proposed for these loci.) Originally, the D loci specificities were identified by MLC, and antigens recognized by serological tissue typing which appeared to be due to the same molecules were termed 'DR' (D-related). However, SB and DC loci also contribute to MLC HLA-D reactivity.

MB and MT are a group of serologically detected determinants associated with the HLA-D region molecules.

HLA class 3 molecules are encoded in a section of the chromosome between HLA-B and HLA-D. They include the C2 and B genes and the pseudoalleles for C4, C4F and C4S, which are also the Rogers and Chido blood groups respectively.

Pseudoalleles / Tandem alleles are gene loci found closely together and encoding the same type of protein, so that two variants are present on the same haplotype.

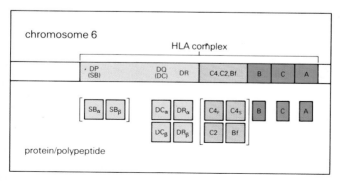

Fig.4.4 The human MHC.

H-2 HAPLOTYPES

The table below lists some of the most commonly used inbred strains, along with their H-2 haplotype. The haplotypes of the cell surface markers of the Qa, Tla, Ly1, Ly2/3 and Thy loci, which encode cell surface molecules on T lymphocytes, are also shown. The Igh-C haplotypes refer to those genes which encode the constant portion of the Igδ heavy chains. ('•' = not determined.) The H-2 haplotypes are designated by small superscripted letters, for example, A/J mice are H-2^a and AKR mice are H-2^k etc.

strain	chromosomes and gene locus						
	17			9	19	6	12
	H-2	Qa1,2,3	Tla	Thy 1	Ly 1,	2/3	Igh-C
A/J	a	a a a	a	b	b	bb	e
AKR	k	b b b	b	a	b	aa	d
BALB/c	d	b a a	c	b	b	bb	a
CBA/Ca	k	. b b	b	b	a	ab	j
C3H/He	k	b b b	b	b	a	ab	j
C57BL/6	b	b a a	b	b	b	bb	b
C57BL/10	b	. a a	b	•	b	bb	b
C58	k	a b b	a	b	b	aa	•
DBA1	q	b a b	b	b	a	ab	c
DBA2	d	b a a	c	b	a	ab	c
NZB	d	a a a	a	b	b	bb	n
NZW	z	. b b	•	•	•	• •	n
SJL	s	a . .	a	b	b	bb	b
129	b	a a a	c	b	b	bb	a

Fig.4.5 Haplotypes of inbred mouse strains.

bm mutants are strains of mice which were derived from an H-2^b strain and which developed mutations in the H-2 region. Mice with such mutations in the H-2 region designated H-2^{bm} induce graft rejection reactions in H-2^b mice. The majority of these mutations occur in the H-2K molecule.

The table below lists some of the more common mouse strains derived from single or double recombinations in the H-2 region. The point at which the recombination occurred was defined by genetic analyses which generally have not yet been identified in the DNA sequence. Haplotype nomenclature is similar to that described above, so for example, the strain A.TL is H-2K^s, H-2I^k and H-2D^d.

		H-2 recombinant strains					
DNA map	K	I-A			I-E		S	D
gene locus	K	I-A	I-B	I-J	I-E	I-C	S	D
strain								
A.AL	k	k	k	k	k	k	k	d
A.TL	s	k	k	k	k	k	k	d
B10.A(2R)	k	k	k	k	k	d	d	b
B10.A(3R)	b	b	b	b	k	d	d	d
B10.A(4R)	k	k	b	b	b	b	b	b
B10.A(5R)	b	b	b	k	k	d	d	d
B10.AQR	q	k	k	k	d	d	d	d
B10.HTG	d	d	d	d	d	d	d	b
B10.MBR	b	k	k	k	k	k	k	q
B10.AKM	k	k	k	k	k	k	k	q
B10.T(6R)	q	q	q	q	q	q	q	d
ATH.B10.S(7R)	s	s	s	s	s	s	s	d

Fig.4.6 Haplotypes of H-2 recombinant strains.

MHC TYPING

Tissue typing is the technique used to determine the MHC specificities carried on an individual's cells. There are two main ways of doing this, either serologically or by MLC. Since MHC molecules occur on the cell surface they can be recognized as antigens by allogeneically different individuals, and antisera can be raised to them. Typing is performed by adding antisera of defined specificity (eg. anti-HLA B8) to the cell to be typed (usually lymphocytes). Addition of complement kills the cells and this can be visualized by staining with trypan blue which is taken up by dead cells (Fig.4.7 right).

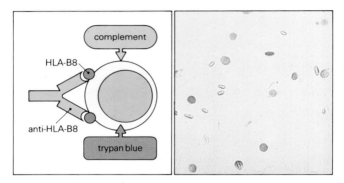

Fig.4.7 Tissue typing - serological.

Typing sera, specific for particular MHC molecules, are obtained by immunizing allogeneic individuals with cells and absorbing out unwanted antibodies to make the sera totally specific for the required MHC determinant. Monoclonal antibodies to some determinants are now available. Sera are also obtained from individuals who have become sensitised to, and subsequently rejected an allogeneic graft or from women who have become sensitized to foetal MHC antigens during their pregnancy.

Public (supratypic) and Private specificities. Antibodies raised against framework parts of MHC molecules often cross-react with several MHC antigens; these recognize public specificities, whereas antibodies which bind to only one MHC molecule are said to recognize private specificities.

Mixed Lymphocyte Culture/Reaction (MLC/MLR) is a technique for typing cells, in which lymphocytes of different individuals are cocultured. If the cells differ they are stimulated

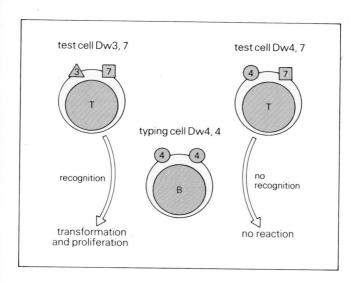

Fig.4.8 Tissue typing - Mixed Lymphocyte Reaction.

to divide. The test can either be performed where each set of cells can react to the other (two way MLC) or where one set (stimulator) is treated so it cannot respond and only the proliferation of the responding (test) cells is measured (one way MLC). In the example above, the test cell Dw 3,7 reacts to the stimulator (typing) cell Dw 4,4 but the test cell Dw 4,7 shares a haplotype with the typing cell and does not respond. Therefore, lack of response indicates that the test cell and typing cell share a specificity.

Homozygous Typing cells are cells with two identical MHC haplotypes. Human typing cells often come from offspring of first cousin marriages.

Lymphocyte activating determinants (Lads) are the cell surface determinants which induce MLC stimulation. MHC class 2 molecules are primarily responsible.

Primed Lymphocyte Test (PLT). This is a highly sensitive MLC assay for detecting Lads in which the test cells are mixed with lymphocytes which were previously primed to a particular Lad by homozygous typing cells. The primed cells proliferate rapidly if the test cell carries the Lad of the original homozygous priming cell. In this procedure it is the primed cells, not the test cells, which proliferate.

MHC FUNCTIONS

MHC restriction. The MHC controls interactions between cells of the immune system, where the cells must share an MHC region (or subregion) to cooperate optimally. These types of interaction (illustrated opposite) are said to be MHC restricted. (See also 'genetic restriction' and 'class 1/2 restriction'.)

1) Antigen-presenting cells (APC) present antigen (Ag) to helper T cells (T_H) in association with MHC class 2 molecules (Ia). Receptors on the T cell recognize antigen (Ag^r) and Ia (Ia^r). The Ia receptor may in part consist of the T4 cell surface marker or its equivalent, which is present on class 2 restricted cells.

2) Some antigen-specific factors released by T cells help B cells of the same MHC type. These factors can bind to APCs in association with antigen; B cells then recognize the matrix of antigen and factor via their surface immunoglobulin (Ig) and Ia. Further proliferation signals (eg. IL-1) may come from the APC. Some helper factors appear to contain I region encoded determinants which could also lead to class 2 restriction.

3) T cells help B cells directly across an antigen bridge - in an MHC class 2 restricted interaction. It is probable that the basis of this interaction is the recognition by the T cell of Ia/antigen determinants on the B cell.

4) Cytotoxic reactions include the killing of virally-infected targets and the graft rejection reactions which originally identified the MHC. T_H cells recognize viral antigen and class 2 molecules, either on the target cell or on an APC. They then deliver help to cytotoxic T cells (Tc), which recognize antigen in association with class 1 molecules (possibly via a receptor which includes the T8 molecule). These signals trigger the Tc cell to kill the target. In graft rejection, the foreign MHC antigens on the target are by themselves equivalent to the MHC- plus-Ag signal required to activate T cells. Lymphokines released by activated cells recruit macrophages, which may also damage the graft.

5) T suppressor cells (Ts) release factors which interact in an IJ-restricted fashion to suppress the activity of T and B cells. The factors may act by binding to antigen-presenting cells, but as suggested for the action of T helper factors above, the molecular basis of this finding has not been clearly determined. Some suppressor factors appear to carry determinants which are recognized by allogeneic anti-IJ region antisera, in addition to an antigen specific portion.

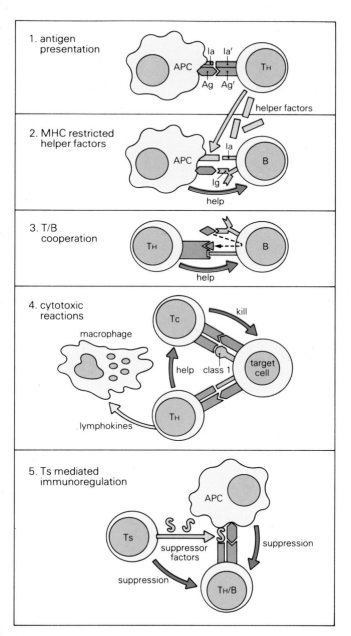

Fig.4.9 Summary of MHC restricted reactions.

EDUCATION OF T CELLS

Education of T cells. This is the process in which T cells learn to recognize antigen in association with self-MHC molecules, so that subsequently they can only be activated by antigens associated with the same MHC. Evidence for this was adduced using radiation chimaeras.

Chimaeras are animals containing cells of different genotypes. Radiation chimaeras are produced by lethally irradiating an animal and reconstituting it with haemopoietic cells of an allogeneically different strain of that species.

Thymic education is the theory that pre-T cells developing in the thymus interact with thymic epithelium, and on maturation only recognize antigen on cells which have the same haplotype as that thymus. Evidence for this view is presented in the table below. In the experiment recipient mice are irradiated and reconstituted with donor bone marrow cells. They are then infected with virus and their lymphocytes tested for cytotoxicity against virally-infected targets of type A or B. If donor AxB cells mature in an A or B recipient, they kill only targets of the recipient type (1 & 2). If the recipient is also thymectomized and given a thymus graft, the recipient can now only kill cells with the same haplotype as the thymus (3 & 4), indicating that the haplotype of the recipient thymus is critical. Experiments such as these which use chimaeras pose many problems due to: 1) some of the recipient's immunocompetent cells survive in some radiation chimaeras, 2) many systems do not differentiate the role of MHC restriction in thymic education and antigen presentation and 3) not all chimaeras are stable and so GvH reactions can occur.

	donor bone marrow	recipient (irradiated)	recipient thymus	killing of target cells of:	
				type A	type B
1.	AxB	A	A	+	−
2.	AxB	B	B	−	+
3.	AxB	thymectomized AxB	A graft	+	−
4.	AxB	thymectomized AxB	B graft	−	+

Fig.4.10 Thymic education of cytotoxic T cells.

TRANSPLANTATION

Tissue transplants and immune reactions between cells of different individuals can be divided according to the donor/recipient combination as follows:

Xenogeneic/xenografts describe immune reactions or tissue grafting between different species,
Allogeneic/allografts are reactions or grafts between genetically non-identical members of the same species,
Syngeneic/isografts are between genetically identical individuals, and
Autografts are made with the recipient's own tissues.

Laws of transplantation state that grafts will be accepted if the recipient shares certain genes (histocompatibility genes) with the graft donor. So in the examples below, a strain A mouse accepts a strain A graft but not a strain B graft. The $(A \times B)F_1$ accepts the B graft because it has the B genes, but the B mouse rejects the $(A \times B)F_1$ graft because it lacks the A genes.

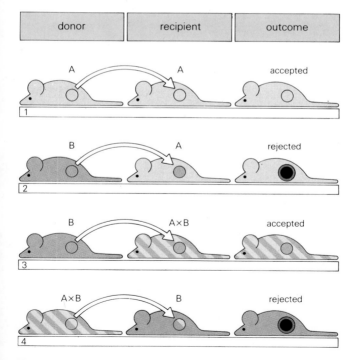

Fig.4.11 The laws of transplantation.

Histocompatibility concerns the ability of an individual to accept grafts from another individual.

Histocompatibility genes. These determine whether a graft is accepted. A large number of gene loci affect graft rejection, but one locus, the Major Histocompatibility Complex, is most important. The MHC was originally identified for this function, but it is now known to have many other roles.

Transplantation antigens are allogeneic cell surface molecules recognized by T cells. MHC class 1 molecules present on all nucleated cells are particularly important.

Minor histocompatibility loci encode antigens which can induce weak graft rejection. There are up to 30 such loci in the mouse, H-1, H-3 etc. (H-2 is the MHC.) Reactions induced by antigens at these loci can usually be suppressed, but MHC-induced reactions often cannot.

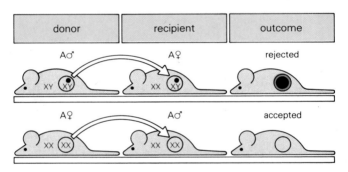

Fig.4.12 The H-Y antigen.

H-Y is a monomorphic histocompatibility antigen encoded on the male (Y) chromosome. When female mice receive grafts from males of the same strain they sometimes recognize the H-Y antigen and reject the graft, whereas the males accept grafts from females.

First and Second set rejection. The immune reactions which produce graft rejection display specificity and memory. For example, a skin allograft in man will normally be rejected in 10 - 14 days (*first set*) but if a second allograft from the same individual (or an individual with the same tissue type) is given, the recipient will reject it more rapidly, usually in 5 - 7 days (*second set*). This accelerated reaction is specific for grafts of the tissue type which first sensitized the recipient.

Rejection reactions are induced by recipient T-helper cells which recognize allogeneic MHC antigens. These can help cytotoxic T cells, which also recognize allogeneic MHC, to kill the target cells. Another possibility is that macrophages recruited to the graft site by lymphokines from the T_H cells, cause the damage. This hypothesis has some similarities to Type IV hypersensitivity reactions.

Passenger cells are donor leucocytes present in the graft tissue. They are thought to be particularly important in sensitizing recipient T-helper cells to donor antigens since they express class 2 MHC molecules, and they can migrate out of the graft into the recipient's lymphatic system.

Crossmatching. To avoid graft rejection the tissue type of the donor and recipient are crossmatched. All donor/recipients are matched for the ABO blood group, and where practical, for as many MHC class 1 and 2 specificities as possible. The greater the number of shared specificities, the higher the chance of graft survival.

Priveleged tissues. Some allogeneic graft tissues induce only weak immune reactions, eg. liver. One explanation is that the priveleged tissues express relatively few MHC antigens on their cell surfaces.

Priveleged sites are areas where implanted grafts are largely isolated from the recipient's immune system. For example, the cornea of the eye lacks a lymphatic drainage, and corneal allografts often do not sensitize the recipient.

Hyperacute/Acute/Chronic rejection describe the speed of rejection in organs such as the kidney. *Hyperacute* reactions occur within minutes of implantation and are caused by preformed recipient antibody to the graft. *Acute* rejection occurs within 2 weeks of grafting, due to prior sensitization of the recipient to histocompatibility antigens. *Chronic* rejection develops later due to the development of sensitivity to graft antigens. This sometimes occurs after the cessation of immunosuppression necessitated by infection.

Graft versus Host disease (GvH) is a condition where immunocompetent donor cells (eg. from a bone marrow graft) recognize and react against the recipient's tissues, either because the recipient is immunosuppressed or cannot recognize the allogeneic cells. Sensitized donor T-helper cells can recruit the recipient's macrophages to organs to cause pathological damage. The skin, gut epithelium and liver are most frequently affected.

5 Inflammation and Phagocytosis

INFLAMMATION

Inflammation is the response of tissue to injury, with the function of bringing serum molecules and cells of the immune system to the site of damage. The reaction consists of three components. 1) Increased blood supply to the region. 2) Increased capillary permeability in the affected area. 3) Emigration of cells out of the blood vessels and into the tissues.

Vasodilation is the dilation of the local blood vessels caused by the action of mediators on the smooth muscle of the vessel walls, producing increased blood flow.

Transudate/Exudate. Normally only small molecules pass freely through the capillary wall, while larger proteins are retained in the plasma. The fluid which passes through is a

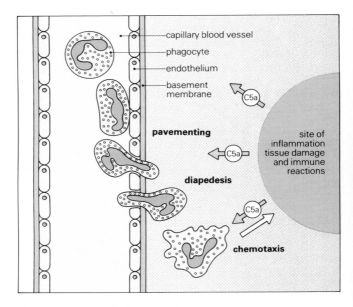

Fig.5.1 **Stages of chemotaxis.**

transudate. If inflammation occurs the endothelial cells are caused to retract, permitting large molecules to pass out. This fluid, which is also rich in cells, is an inflammatory *exudate*.

Pavementing and Diapedesis are the stages by which neutrophils and macrophages emigrate from the blood stream. The cells first adhere to the capillary endothelium (pavementing) and then extend pseudopodia between the endothelial cells, dissolve the basement membrane and migrate out into the tissues (diapedesis).

Chemotaxis is directional movement in response to an inflammatory mediator. Cells appear to migrate up concentration gradients of chemotactic molecules, such as C5a.

Chemokinesis is increased random (ie non-directional) movement of cells caused by a biochemical mediator.

Acute phase proteins are molecules whose serum concentration increases during infection, eg CRP.

C-Reactive Protein (CRP), a molecule which reacts with the C polysaccharide of pneumococci and acts as an opsonin.

Interferons (IFN) are a group of molecules which limit the spread of viral infection. There are three types, IFNα and IFNβ, produced by leucocytes and fibroblasts, and IFNγ, produced by activated T cells. Interferons from activated or virally-infected cells bind to receptors on nearby cells, inducing these cells to make anti-viral proteins. IFNγ also modulates immune responses and enhances NK cell activity.

Anti-viral proteins induced by interferon are molecules which prevent viral replication. Some, which are activated by virus, interfere with protein synthesis.

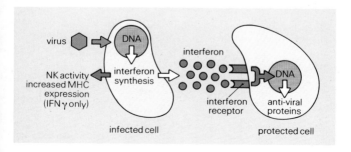

Fig.5.2 The action of interferon.

Inflammation is mediated by a variety of molecules derived from the plasma enzyme systems, cells of the immune system, mast cells and from the pathogens themselves. The

mediator	origin	actions
histamine	mast cells basophils	increased vascular permeability smooth muscle contraction chemokinesis
5-hydroxy tryptamine (5HT) = serotonin	platelets mast cells (rodents)	increased vascular permeability smooth muscle contraction
platelet activating factor (PAF)	basophils neutrophils macrophages	mediator release from platelets increased vascular permeability smooth muscle contraction neutrophil activation
neutrophil chemotactic factor (NCF)	mast cells	neutrophil chemotaxis
C3a	complement C3	mast cell degranulation smooth muscle contraction
C5a	complement C5	mast cell degranulation neutrophil and macrophage chemotaxis, neutrophil activation smooth muscle contraction increased capillary permeability
bradykinin	kinin system (kininogen)	vasodilation smooth muscle contraction increased vascular permeability pain
fibrinopeptides and fibrin break-down products	clotting system	increased vascular permeability neutrophil and macrophage chemotaxis
prostaglandin E_2 (PGE_2)	cyclooxygenase pathway	vasodilation potentiate increased vascular permeability produced by histamine and bradykinin
leukotriene B4 (LTB_4)	lipoxygenase pathway	neutrophil chemotaxis synergises with PGE_2 in increasing vascular permeability
leukotriene D4 (LTD_4)	lipoxygenase pathway	smooth muscle contraction increased vascular permeability

Fig.5.3 Mediators of acute inflammation.

mediators are listed opposite and the diagram below indicates how the various systems interact to generate the mediators.

Kinins are generated following tissue injury. Bradykinin is the most important. It is produced by the action of kallikrein on kininogen. Kallikrein results from the action of Hageman factor on prekallikrein, or via enzymes from damaged tissues.

Eicosanoids are inflammatory mediators produced from arachidonic acid, which is released from membranes by the action of phospholipase A2. Arachidonic acid is converted into eicosanoids by mast cells and macrophages via two major pathways (cyclooxygenase and lipoxygenase pathways).

Prostaglandins (PG) and Thromboxanes (Tx) are produced by the action of cyclooxygenase on arachidonic acid. Prostaglandins and thromboxanes enhance or inhibit inflammation depending on the mediator and its level.

Leukotrienes are produced by the lipoxygenase pathway which generates mediators of acute inflammation and the slow reacting substances important in hypersensitivity.

Formyl-methionyl peptides (fMet-) are bacterial products which are highly chemotactic for neutrophils.

Endogenous pyrogen is interleukin 1 (IL-1). It causes fever and induces prostaglandin production.

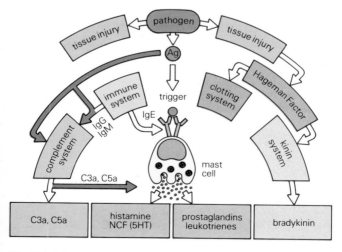

Fig.5.4 Plasma enzyme systems.

PHAGOCYTOSIS

Phagocytosis is the process by which cells engulf particles and microorganisms. The particles first attach to the cell membrane of the phagocytic cell, either by non-specific receptors, or by receptors for opsonins such as IgG and C3b. Then the cell extends pseudopodia around the particle and internalizes it. Lysosomes then fuse with the phagosome. The lysosomal enzymes damage and digest the phagocytosed material and digestion products are finally released.

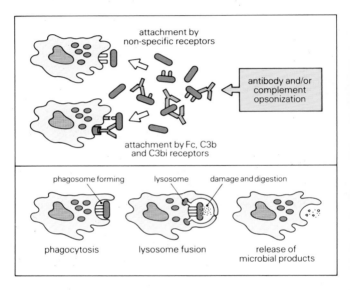

Fig.5.5 Stages of phagocytosis.

Pinocytosis is phagocytosis on a small scale in which cells take up small volumes of extracellular fluid.

Opsonization occurs when particles, micoorganisms or immune complexes become coated with molecules which make them more easily phagocytosed.

Opsonins are molecules which bind both to particles to be phagocytosed and to receptors on phagocytic cells, so acting as a bridge between the two. Examples are IgG, C3b and CRP.

Immune adherence refers to the attachment of opsonized particles to phagocytes, effected by IgG and C3 products.

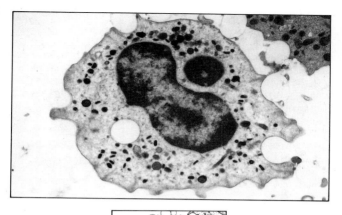

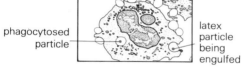

phagocytosed particle —

latex particle being engulfed

Fig.5.6 Phagocytosis of latex by a macrophage.

Complement Receptors (CR). There are three different kinds of receptor for activated C3 (C3b, C3bi and C3d). Different cells have different sets of receptors. The receptors are not totally specific for each molecule.

CR1 (C3b receptor) occurs on neutrophils, eosinophils, monocytes, macrophages, B cells, some T cells and erythrocytes. It binds to C3b, C3bi and C4b. On phagocytes it facilitates attachment to particles but its role on lymphocytes is uncertain.

CR2 (C3d receptor) is present on B lymphocytes. It binds to C3d and more weakly to C3b and C3bi, and it may be involved in the development of B cell memory.

CR3 (C3bi receptor) is expressed on neutrophils and monocytes. It binds to C3b which has been cleaved by factor I. It functions in phagocyte attachment.

Frustrated phagocytosis occurs when phagocytes attach to material which cannot be phagocytosed (eg. basement membrane). The cells may release their lysosomal enzymes to the exterior (exocytosis). This process is thought to cause some of the damage in immune complex disease.

Phagosomes are the membrane bound intracellular vesicles which contain phagocytosed materials.

Oxygen-dependent killing occurs within the phagosomes. Initially an enzyme in the phagosome membrane, possibly an oxidase or cytochrome B, reduces oxygen to superoxide (O_2^-) which can then give rise to hydroxyl radicals (OH^-), singlet oxygen ($O^.$) and hydrogen peroxide (H_2O_2), all of which can damage bacteria.

Peroxidase present in lysosomes can enter the phagosome where, in the presence of H_2O_2, it converts halide ions into toxic halogen compounds (eg. hypohalite). Endocytosed peroxidase or catalase can also perform this reaction.

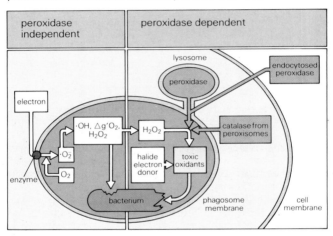

Fig.5.7 Oxygen-dependent microbicidal activity.

Respiratory burst. Shortly after phagocytosing material neutrophils undergo a burst of activity. During this time the cells increase their oxygen consumption. This is associated with increased activity of the hexose monophosphate shunt and production of H_2O_2 and O_2^-.

Chemiluminescence is the production of light by chemical reactions. It occurs during the respiratory burst.

Lysosomes are organelles present in all cells. They contain enzymes, which in macrophages, damage and digest the phagocytosed material. Newly forming lysosomes are called 'primary', and mature lysosomes are 'secondary'.

Phagolysosomes are formed by the fusion of phagosomes and lysosomes. Immediately after phagosome/lysosome fusion there is a brief rise in the pH of the phagolysosome, and neutral proteases and cationic proteins are active. Subsequently the pH falls and acid proteases become active.

Granules are specialized lysosomes of granulocytes, which contain various bactericidal proteins. Each type of granule has a particular set of proteins. For example, neutrophil myeloperoxidase is in the primary (azurophilic) granules whereas lactoferrin is in the secondary (neutrophil specific) granules.

Granule and lysosome contents include:
Lysozyme (muramidase), an enzyme which digests a bond in the cell wall proteoglycan of some gram-positive bacteria. It is secreted by neutrophils and some macrophages and is present in many of the body's secretions.

Cationic proteins found in neutrophil granules and in some macrophages damage the outer lipid bilayer of some gram-negative bacteria under alkaline conditions. This activity is produced by a number of molecules, some of which (eg. cathepsin G) are enzymically active.

Acid proteases, active at acid pH, include enzymes such as glycosidase, nuclease, lipase and acid phosphatase.

Neutral proteases, active near pH 7, include enzymes such as collagenase, elastase and some cathepsins.

Lactoferrin, found in neutrophil granules, binds tightly to iron, thus depriving bacteria of this essential molecule. Neutrophils loaded with iron are inefficient at destroying bacteria.

Macrophage activation refers to the enhanced anti-microbial (or anti-tumour) activity seen in response to stimulation by lymphokines, complement fragments etc. Activated cells secrete more enzymes, produce more superoxide and express more Fc and C3b receptors.

Chediak-Higashi syndrome is a condition with impaired phagocyte responses to chemoattractants and reduced killing of phagocytosed bacteria. The primary disorder appears to lie in the cells' cytoskeletal system.

Chronic Granulomatous Disease (CGD) is a genetic defect where oxygen-dependent bacterial killing is impaired and mononuclear cells accumulate at sites of chronic infection, forming granulomas.

COMPLEMENT

Complement is one of the serum enzyme systems. Its functions include mediating inflammation, opsonization of antigenic particles (including microorganisms) and causing membrane damage to pathogens. The system consists of 19 separate proteins which may be activated either via the 'classical' or 'alternative' pathways. Molecules of the classical pathway are designated C1,C2 etc. Alternative pathway molecules have letter designations, for example, factor B (or FB, or just B), factor D etc. The physicochemical properties and functions of the complement components are given overleaf and their reactions are shown opposite.

Enzyme cascade. The complement components interact with each other so that the products of one reaction form the enzyme for the next, thus a small initial stimulus can trigger an increasing cascade of activity. Small fragments of complements molecules produced by cleavage are subscripted 'a' (C3a, Ba etc) and large fragments 'b' (C3b, Bb etc). Active enzymes are designated by a bar, for example, $\overline{C3b}$, $\overline{Bb}$ etc).

The classical pathway (backshaded yellow) is activated by immune complexes binding to C1, via the C1q subcomponent which has 6 Fc binding sites. This induces enzymic cleavage of C1r and C1s. $\overline{C1s}$ then splits C4a from C4 and C2a from C2, leaving $\overline{C4b2b}$ which can then cleave C3.

The alternative pathway (properdin pathway or amplification loop) (backshaded purple) is activated in the presence of suitable surfaces or molecules, including microbial products. C3b can either bind H or B. Normally H is bound and C3b is inactivated by I, but in the presence of activators B is bound which is then enzymically cleaved by D releasing Ba and leaving $\overline{C3b,Bb}$ an enzyme which can cleave C3. This gives a positive feedback (amplification) loop to generate more C3b.

C3-convertases, including $\overline{C4b2b}$ ($\overline{C4b2a}$ in WHO nomenclature) and $\overline{C3b,Bb}$, clip C3a from C3 to leave C3b. C3b has a labile binding site which allows it to covalently bind to nearby molecules. C3b together with a C3-convertase can cleave C5.

The lytic pathway (backshaded orange) is activated when C5b is deposited on membranes. C5b associates with C6,C7,C8 and C9 to form the membrane attack complex.

Membrane attack complex (MAC) is a structure of C5b678 and polymeric C9 which traverses the target cell membrane and allows osmotic leakage from the cell.

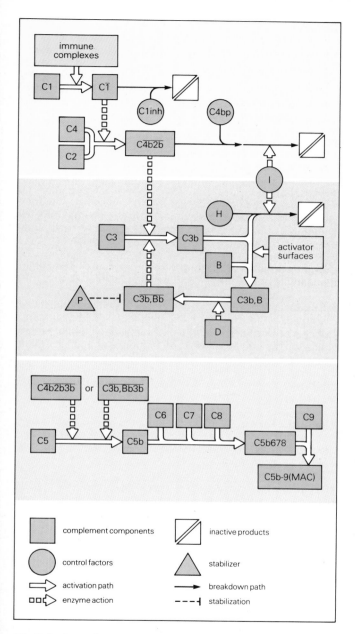

Fig.5.8 Complement reaction pathways.

Complement fixation is the activation of complement followed by deposition of the activated components on nearby immune complexes or cell membranes. Following activation of C4b, C3b and C5b a highly reactive group is exposed which can form ester links with OH groups. The reactive group decays quickly by hydrolysis if a link is not formed. For this reason complement components only deposit close to the site at which they were activated.

Bystander lysis is the phenomenon where cells in close proximity to a site of complement activation have active components deposited on them and are then lysed.

Anaphylatoxins. C3a and C5a mediate inflammation by causing mast cell degranulation, smooth muscle contraction and increased capillary permeability following retraction of endothelial cells. In this way they mimic some of the reactions of anaphylaxis.

Conglutinin is a naturally occurring molecule in species of ruminants which binds to C3bi.

Immunoconglutinin is an autoantibody which binds C3b.

Cobra Venom Factor (CVF) is a molecule in cobra venom which can be used experimentally to deplete an animal of C3. It is in fact cobra C3b which binds to B and can form a C3-convertase, (CVF,Bb) but it is not susceptible to the normal regulatory inactivation by H and I, so it produces uncontrolled C3 activation.

Nephritic Factor (NeF) is an autoantibody found in high concentrations in some kidney diseases which binds to, and stabilizes C3b,Bb, thus potentiating alternative pathway activity (cf. properdin).

Hereditary angioedema is a condition caused by genetic deficiency of C1inh, in which there is uncontrolled local activation of C2, which then undergoes conversion into C2 kinin, a pathological oedema-producing peptide.

Paroxysmal Nocturnal Haemoglobinuria (PNH) is a condition in which there is red cell breakdown. This is due to the patient's red cells activating the alternative pathway. The red cells have low levels of membrane sialic acid, and act as an activator surface.

Zymosan is a component of yeast cell walls which is a potent activator of the alternative pathway.

component	mol. wt. (KD)	serum conc. (µg/ml)	no. of polypeptides	function
C1q	410	150	18	form a Ca^{++} linked complex – C1q C1r$_2$ C1s$_2$; C1q binds to complexed Ig to activate the classical pathway
C1r	83	50	1	
C1s	83	50	1	
C4	210	550	3	classical pathway molecules, activated by C1s to form a C3 convertase, $\overline{C4b2b}$
C2	115	25	1	
C3	180	1200	2	active C3 (C3b) opsonizes anything to which it binds and activates the lytic pathway. C3a causes mast cell degranulation and smooth muscle contraction. C3bi, C3d, C3e and C3g are breakdown products of C3b
C5	180	70	2	C5b on membranes initiates the lytic pathway. C5a is chemotactic for macrophages and neutrophils, causes smooth muscle contraction, mast cell degranulation and increased capillary permeability
C6	130	60	1	lytic pathway components which assemble in the presence of C5b to form the membrane attack complex and so may cause cell lysis
C7	120	50	1	
C8	155	55	3	
C9	75	60	1	
B	95	200	1	B binds to C3b in the presence of alternative pathway activators. It is then cleaved by D, an active serum enzyme to form a C3 convertase $\overline{C3b,Bb}$
D	25	10	1	
P (properdin)	185	25	4	stabilizes $\overline{C3b,Bb}$ to potentiate amplification loop activity
C4bp	550	250	8	C4bp binds C4b and H binds to C3b, to act as cofactors for I which cleaves and inactivates C3b and C4b
H (β_1H)	150	500	1	
I (C3bina)	100	30	2	
C1 inh	100	185	1	binds and inactivates $\overline{C1r_2}$ and $\overline{C1s_2}$

Fig.5.9 **The complement components.**

6 Immunopathology

HYPERSENSITIVITY

Hypersensitivity describes an immune response which occurs in an exaggerated or inappropriate form. These reactions have been classified into four major types by Gell and Coombs, according to the speed of the reaction and the immune mechanisms involved. Although they are classified

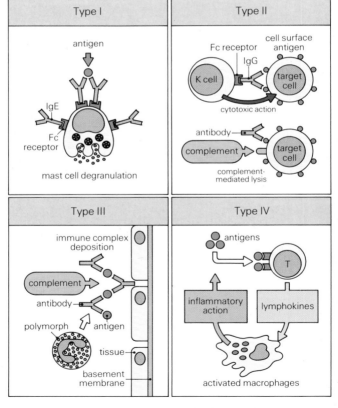

Fig.6.1 Four types of hypersensitivity reaction.

separately, in practice they do not necessarily occur in isolation from each other. Furthermore, several different immune reactions may be subsumed in a single type.

Type I (Immediate) hypersensitivity which is manifested in allergic asthma, hay fever and excema develops within minutes of exposure to antigen. It is dependent on the activation of mast cells and the release of mediators of acute inflammation. Mast cells bind IgE via their surface Fc$^\epsilon$ receptors and when antigen crosslinks the IgE the mast cells degranulate, releasing vasoactive amines, which produce inflammation. Prostaglandins and leukotrienes produced by arachidonic acid metabolism, contribute to a delayed component of the reaction which often develops several hours after the original antigen exposure.

Type II (Antibody-mediated) hypersensitivity is caused by antibody to cell surface antigens. These can sensitize the cells for antibody-dependent cell-mediated cytotoxicity by K cells, or complement mediated lysis. Type II hypersensitivity is seen in the destruction of red blood cells in transfusion reactions, and in haemolytic disease of the newborn. The destruction of tissue in autoimmune diseases such as myasthenia gravis is also partly antibody-mediated.

Type III (Immune complex mediated) hypersensitivity is due to the deposition of antigen/antibody complexes in tissue and blood vessels. These activate complement and attract polymorphs to the site, causing local damage. The antigens come from persistent pathogenic infections (eg. malaria), from inhaled antigens (eg. extrinsic allergic alveolitis) or from the host's own tissue, in autoimmune diseases. These conditions are all characterized by a high antigen load, which may be associated with a weak or ineffective antibody response.

Type IV (Delayed) hypersensitivity arises more than 24 hours after encounter with the antigen, and is mediated by antigen-sensitized T cells which release lymphokines, attracting macrophages to the site and activating them. The macrophages produce tissue damage which may develop into chronic granulomatous reactions if the antigen persists. This type of hypersensitivity is seen in skin contact reactions and in the response to some chronic pathogens, such as *M. tuberculosis* and *Schistosoma spp*.

Type V (Stimulatory) hypersensitivity describes reactions where autoantibodies stimulate host tissue, such as the stimulation of thyroid by autoantibody binding to the TSH receptor, thus mimicking thyroid stimulating hormone.

TYPE I (IMMEDIATE) HYPERSENSITIVITY

Allergy, originally meaning altered reactivity on second contact with an antigen, is now usually taken to mean a Type I hypersensitivity reaction.

Allergen is an antigen which induces a Type I reaction.

Sensitization in this context is the process by which a susceptible individual develops allergen-specific IgE, which becomes fixed to Fc^ϵ receptors on the mast cell.

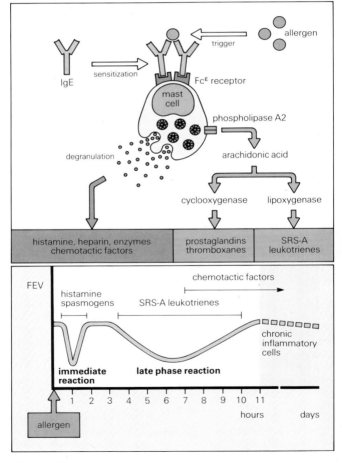

Fig.6.2 Type I hypersensitivity.

Triggering occurs when antigen crosslinks mast cell surface IgE, which causes an influx of Ca^{++}, resulting in degranulation and activation of phospholipase A2.

Degranulation occurs when mast cell granules fuse with the plasma membrane, releasing their contents to the exterior.

Phospholipase A2 is a membrane-associated enzyme which releases arachidonic acid, the initial substrate for the cyclooxygenase and lipoxygenase pathways, which produce prostaglandins and leukotrienes respectively.

Atopy describes conditions which manifest Type I hypersensitivity, including asthma, hay fever and eczema, which tend to cluster in families. These reactions are exemplified below by allergic asthma induced by breathing an allergen.

Immediate and Late phase reactions. Following bronchial provocation with an allergen there is an immediate reduction in airway patency, measured as a fall in forced expiratory volume (FEV), caused by histamine, prostaglandins and via the action of PAF on platelets. After several hours a late phase reaction may ensue, caused by slow reacting substances (SRS) and the accumulation of inflammatory cells, including macrophages, basophils and other polymorphs attracted by chemotactic factors. Analogous immediate and late reactions are seen in skin reactions to topically applied allergens.

SRS-A, originally identified as a mediator of the late phase reaction, consists of leukotrienes C4 and B4.

Anaphylaxis is an immediate systemic Type I hypersensitivity reaction seen in sensitized animals injected with the allergen. The release of vasoactive amines and spasmogens causes smooth muscle contraction and increased vascular permeability with a fall in blood pressure, which can produce respiratory or circulatory failure.

Passive Cutaneous Anaphylaxis (PCA) is an assay for antigen-specific IgE in which an animal is sensitized by passive subcutaneous injection of test serum and then challenged with allergen. If specific IgE is present in the test serum the local mast cells degranulate, releasing histamine and increasing vascular permeability. This is measured by the extravasation of a dye (Evans blue).

Prausnitz Kustner reaction is the equivalent to PCA performed on humans. The positive reaction gives a wheal at the injection site, rather than extravasation of injected dye.

TYPE II (ANTIBODY-MEDIATED) HYPERSENSITIVITY

Type II hypersensitivity is caused by antibody directed to membranes and cell surface antigens. Effector cells with Fc receptors engage the sensitized target. Activation of complement C3 can lead to cell lysis and deposited C3 is recognized by cells with C3 receptors. The site of damage depends on the antibodies involved.

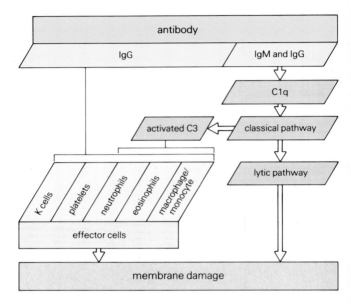

Fig.6.3 Type II hypersensitivity.

Transfusion reactions occur when mismatched donor blood is infused into a recipient. The recipient may have naturally occurring antibodies to the foreign cells, as happens with the ABO blood group system, or they may develop after infusion. The antibodies can cause complement-dependent lysis, or sequestration of the cells.

Blood groups are systems of allotypically variable red blood cell surface antigens, some of which occur on other tissues. The more common ones are listed opposite.

Chido and Rogers blood group antigens are the electrophoretically slow and fast allotypes respectively, of human C4 which have adsorbed to the red cell surface.

system	gene loci	antigens	phenotype frequencies	
ABO	1	A, B or O	A B AB O	42% 8% 3% 47%
Rhesus	3 closely linked loci: major antigen=RhD	C or c D or d E or e	RhD$^+$ RhD$^-$	85% 15%
Kell	1	K or k	K k	9% 91%
Duffy	1	Fy^a, Fy^b or Fy	Fy^{a}Fy^b Fy^a Fy^b Fy	46% 20% 34% 0.1%
MN	1	M or N	MM NN MN	28% 50% 22%

Fig.6.4 Five major human blood group systems.

Haemolytic Disease of the Newborn (HDNB) is caused by maternal antibodies to the foetal red cells which cross the placenta and destroy them. The mother becomes sensitized by foetal red cells entering her circulation at birth, so that the first child is usually unaffected. The most common cases involve Rhesus-negative mothers carrying Rhesus-positive children.

Rhesus prophylaxis is the administration of anti-Rhesus D antibody to Rhesus-negative mothers immediately after delivering a Rhesus-positive child in order to destroy the Rh$^+$ cells and thus prevent them sensitizing the mother.

Autoimmune haemolytic anaemia is caused by auto-antibodies to red cells producing cell destruction by lysis or sequestration. The antibodies responsible are of two types:

Warm agglutinins react with red cells at 37°C.

Cold agglutinins react only below 37°C and therefore tend to bind to red cells in the periphery only.

Goodpastures syndrome: a Type II reaction in which auto-antibodies damage lung and kidney basement membrane.

TYPE III (IMMUNE COMPLEX MEDIATED) HYPERSENSITIVITY

Immune complex deposition. Type III hypersensitivity results from the deposition of immune complexes in blood vessel walls and tissues. Complexes can activate platelets (in humans) and basophils, via Fc receptors, to release vasoactive amines which cause endothelial cell retraction and increased vascular permeability leading to complex deposition. Complexes also activate complement, releasing C3a and C5a. Both of these activate basophils, while C5a also increases vascular permeability and is chemotactic for polymorphs. Polymorphs which fail in the attempt to phagocytose the deposited complexes, release their granules to the exterior, causing local tissue damage. Complexes tend to deposit at sites of high pressure, filtration or turbulence, such as in the kidney or at the bifurcation of arteries.

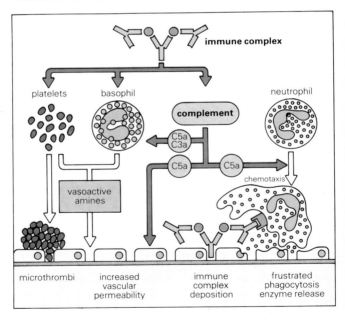

Fig.6.5 Immune complex deposition.

Immune complex clearance, the removal of complexes, is normally effected by cells of the reticuloendothelial system. The factors which affect clearance include:
a) the size of complexes, b) the class and affinity of the

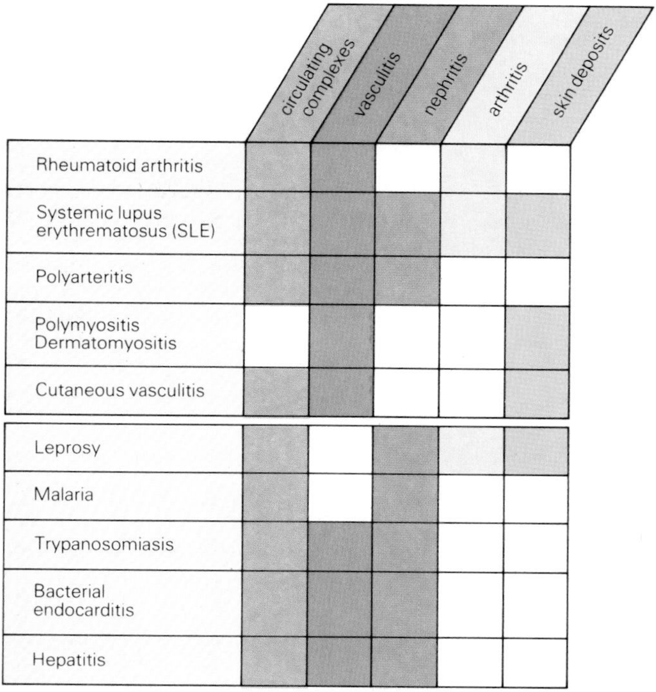

Fig. 6.6 Immune complex diseases: sites of deposition.

	circulating complexes	vasculitis	nephritis	arthritis	skin deposits
Rheumatoid arthritis	■	■		■	
Systemic lupus erythematosus (SLE)	■	■	■	■	■
Polyarteritis	■	■	■		
Polymyositis Dermatomyositis		■			■
Cutaneous vasculitis	■	■			■
Leprosy	■		■		■
Malaria	■		■		
Trypanosomiasis	■	■	■		
Bacterial endocarditis	■	■	■		
Hepatitis	■	■	■		

antibody, c) the valency of the antigen and d) the amount of complexes. This last factor explains why immune complex disease occurs in infections which release large amounts of antigen, and in autoimmune disease where there is a ready supply of autoantigen.

Immune complex diseases result when excessive immune complex deposition occurs in particular organs.

Serum sickness is a Type III reaction which occurs in individuals injected with foreign serum. Antibodies are made to the serum antigens and there is massive immune complex formation, producing nephritis and arteritis.

Arthus reaction is a skin reaction seen as an area of redness and swelling which is maximal 5 - 6 hours after intradermal injection of antigen. It is caused by IgG binding to the injected antigen and triggering inflammation by Type III mechanisms.

TYPE IV (DELAYED) HYPERSENSITIVITY (DTH)

This includes a number of reactions which are maximal at more than 12 hours following challenge with the antigen and which are dependent on antigen-reactive cells, rather than antibody. Reactivity can be transferred with spleen cells, but not with serum; the cell responsible is the T-delayed hypersensitivity (T_D) cell. This cell type is described according to its function and usually T_D cells are found to carry the surface markers of T-helper cells.

Migration Inhibition Test (MIT). This test detects antigen-sensitized T cells. The lymphocytes to be tested are packed together with monocytes and antigen in capillary tubes by centrifugation. The tubes are then cultured on agar plates. If antigen-sensitive T cells are present they release lymphokines (Migration Inhibition Factor) which inhibit the emigration of monocytes from the tubes.

There are four main types of reaction, but they may occur concommitantly or sequentially in the reaction to a particular antigen. For example, if an antigen stimulus persists a tuberculin-type reaction may develop into a Type IV granuloma.

type	Jones-Mote	contact	tuberculin	granulomatous
reaction time	24 hours	48 hours	48 hours	4 weeks
clinical appearance	skin swelling	eczema	local induration and swelling ± fever	skin induration
histological appearance	basophils, lymphocytes, mononuclear cells	mononuclear cells, oedema, raised epidermis	mononuclear cells, lymphocytes and monocytes, reduced macrophages	epithelioid cell granuloma, giant cells, macrophages, fibrosis, ± necrosis
antigen	intradermal antigen eg. ovalbumin	epidermal: eg. nickel, rubber, poison ivy etc.	dermal: tuberculin, mycobacterial and leishmanial antigens	persistent Ag or Ag/Ab complexes in macrophages or 'non immunological' eg. talcum powder

Fig.6.7 Summary of the important characteristics of the four types of delayed hypersensitivity reaction.

Jones Mote reactions (Cutaneous basophil hypersensitivity) appear within 24 hours of skin challenge with antigen. The area beneath the epidermis becomes infiltrated by basophils over 1-6 days with maximal skin swelling on day 1. The response is thought to be normally regulated by suppressor T cells.

Contact hypersensitivity produces an excematous skin reaction in sensitized humans, which is maximal 48 hours after contact with the allergen. The allergens may be large molecules, or small haptens (eg. nickel) which attach to normal body proteins and modify them so that they become antigenic. The Langerhans recirculating cells pick up these antigens and present them to T lymphocytes in the local lymph nodes. Reactions are characterized by mononuclear cell infiltration with oedema and microvesicle formation in the epidermis. The dermis is also usually infiltrated by an increased number of leucocytes.

Tuberculin-type hypersensitivity was originally seen as a reaction produced by subcutaneous injection of tuberculin in patients with tuberculosis, who responded with fever and a swelling at the site of injection. The term more usually refers to the skin reaction induced by any antigen which is maximal at about 48 hours after challenge and consists of lymphocytes, monocytes and macrophages. If the antigenic stimulus persists a granulomatous reaction may ensue. The tuberculin-type reaction can be induced in a sensitized subject by several non-microbial and microbial antigens.

Granulomatous reactions develop where there is a persistent stimulus which macrophages cannot eliminate. Non-antigenic particles (eg. talc) induce non-immunological granulomas, while persistent pathogens, such as *Mycobacteria spp.* and *Schistosomula spp.* induce immunological granulomas. The lesion consists of a palisade of epithelioid cells and macrophages surrounding the infectious agent, which is in turn surrounded by a cuff of lymphocytes. Collagenous capsules may also develop around some pathogens, due to fibroblast proliferation.

Epithelioid cells are large flattened cells with large amounts of endoplasmic reticulum, seen in granulomas, which are thought to be derived from macrophages, although they have fewer phagosomes than macrophages.

Giant cells are large multinucleated cells seen in some granulomas and are probably derived from the fusion of macrophages or epithelioid cells.

AUTOIMMUNITY

Autoimmunity is the reaction of the immune system against the body's own tissues.

Autoantigens/autoantibodies refer to antigen/antibody systems where antibodies are formed to self molecules.

Autoreactive cells are lymphocytes with receptors for autoantigens. These cells can potentially produce an autoimmune response, but do not necessarily do so.

Forbidden clones. Burnett proposed a theory to explain the way the body is normally tolerant to its own tissue by saying that autoreactive cells were effectively forbidden and so were clonally deleted during embryological development. It is now known that autoreactive B cells are present, but they are not normally active.

T cell bypass. It is now thought that self tolerance is maintained at the level of the T cell—self reactive T cells are clonally aborted or functionally deleted (Fig.6.8, A). It is then proposed that in autoimmune disease, autoreactive B cells become activated by a mechanism which bypasses the tolerant T cells. For example, a cross reactive exogenous antigen binding to a T cell could induce help for an auto reactive B cell (B). Alternatively, polyclonal stimulators such as EB virus (EBV) or lipopolysaccharide (LPS) could stimulate the B cells directly (C).

Autoregulatory failure. The control of some autoreactive cells is thought to depend on T-suppressors (D). If there is a failure of the T suppressors or if autoantigen becomes associated with Ia molecules and preferentially stimulates autoreactive T helper cells, then autoimmunity may result (E).

Autoimmune diseases occur when autoimmune reactions result in pathological tissue damage. In general they are either organ specific or organ non-specific.

Organ-specific autoimmune diseases are primarily directed towards particular tissues, for example, autoantibodies to thyroid in Hashimoto's thyroiditis, or to pancreatic islet cells in autoimmune diabetes. Different types of organ-specific autoimmunity tend to occur together in particular individuals and their relatives.

Organ non-specific autoimmune diseases have antibodies to autoantigens with a wide tissue distribution, such as anti-DNA in systemic lupus erythematosus. These conditions often produce Type III immune complex mediated hypersensitivity reactions.

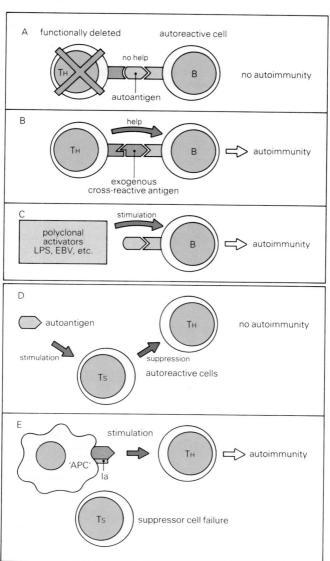

Fig. 6.8 Maintenance and breakdown of self tolerance

IMMUNE DEFICENCIES AND ABNORMALITIES

Immunodeficiency is often identified by the increased frequency of infection in patients. Impaired immunity is a consequence of many pathogenic infections, but primary immunodeficiency is inherited and may affect any part of the immune system, including complement components, granulocytes, macrophages and lymphocytes.

X-linked agammaglobulinaemia (Bruton's disease). Patients with this condition have normal T cell function and cell-mediated immunity to viral infections but have very low immunoglobulin levels and cannot make antibody responses.

Variable hypogammaglobulinaemia patients have low antibody levels but a relatively high incidence of autoimmunity. Usually B cells are present but they fail to differentiate into plasma cells.

DiGeorge syndrome, due to failed development of the 3rd and 4th pharyngeal pouches, results in thymic hypoplasia with low numbera of functionally normal T cells. T cell numbers usually rise to normal levels over 1-2 years.

Severe Combined Immunodeficiency (SCID) is a group of conditions with leucopenia, impaired cell-mediated immunity and low or absent antibody levels. Some cases can be attributed to autosomal recessive adenosine deaminase deficiency or purine nucleoside phosphorylase deficiency. Other cases in which these enzymes are unaffected may be X-linked or autosomal recessive traits.

Acquired Immune Deficiency Syndrome (AIDS) which develops in adults, permits a variety of opportunist infections and is associated with Kaposi's sarcoma. A human T-helper cell cytotropic virus (LAV = HTLV3) is probably the cause.

Thymoma, a thymocyte neoplasia, is associated with immune deficiency and a number of autoimmune diseases, including myasthenia gravis and haemolytic anaemia.

Myeloma (plasmacytoma) are plasma cell tumours which secrete immunoglobulin, usually of limited clonality.

Bence Jones proteins are free light chains present in the urine of some patients with myeloma.

Heavy chain disease is a B lymphocyte disorder where cells produce incomplete Ig heavy chains.

ANIMAL MODELS AND MUTANT STRAINS

The animals listed below have impaired immune systems and are useful for research purposes. Some of the conditions resemble human diseases and therefore are used as models, although it must be emphasized that the resemblance may only be in the *appearance* of the disease. In some cases (eg. nude strains and strains lacking particular receptors) the defect is determined by a single gene locus, but autoimmunity in the autoimmune strains depends on multiple gene loci, which may interact with each other.

Strain/species	Characteristics
Nude mouse Nude rat	The nude mutant (nu) lacks a thymus and all T cells. A linked locus produces hairlessness.
Beige mouse	The beige mutant (bg) has several defects including lack of NK cells.
NZB mouse	Autoimmunity including haemolytic anaemia with failure of immunoregulation.
(NZB/NZW) F_1 mouse	Autoimmunity including immune complex nephritis — possible model of systemic lupus erythematosus.
MRL.lpr	Autoimmunity. The lpr gene produces T cell lymphoproliferation – model of rheumatoid arthritis.
BXSB	Autoimmune, lupus like syndrome with B cell lymphoproliferation.
CBA/n	Lacks a B cell subset (lyb5). Fails to respond to some T-independent antigens.
C3H/HeJ	B cells lack a receptor for LPS.
DBA/2Ha	X-linked defect. B cells lack a receptor for T cell Replacing Factor (TRF).
B/B rat	Spontaneous autoimmune diabetes and thyroid autoimmunity.
Buffalo rat	A proportion develop autoimmune thyroiditis.
Obese chicken	Autoimmune thyroiditis — model of Hashimoto's disease.

Fig.6.9 Characteristics of some immunologically aberrant experimental strains.

7 Immunological Tests and Techniques

ASSAYS FOR ANTIGEN AND ANTIBODY

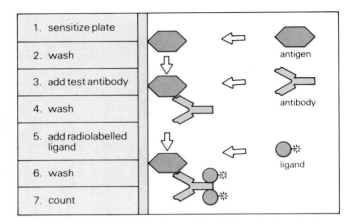

1. sensitize plate
2. wash
3. add test antibody
4. wash
5. add radiolabelled ligand
6. wash
7. count

Fig. 7.1 Radioimmunoassay.

Radioimmunoasay (RIA) includes a variety of techniques which use radiolabelled reagents to detect antigen or antibody. Antibody may be detected using plates sensitized with antigen. Test antibody is applied and this is detected by the addition of a radiolabelled ligand specific for that antibody. The amount of ligand bound to the plate is proportional to the amount of test antibody.

Ligands/Conjugates are made by covalently coupling two molecules together. RIA ligands are usually antibody molecules or protein A, covalently bound to ^{125}I.

Protein A is a cell wall component of Staphylococci which binds specifically to IgG (Fc) of most species.

Radioallergosorbent Test (RAST) is a specialized form of RIA for detecting antigen-specific IgE, in which antigen is covalently coupled to cellulose discs. Antigen-specific IgE binding to the disc is detected using radiolabelled anti-IgE.

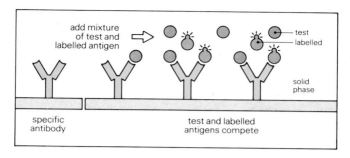

Fig.7.2 Competition Radioimmunoassay.

Competition radioimmunoassay is the classical RIA. It is used to detect antigens. Specific antibody is bound to a solid phase, and a mixture of test (unlabelled) and labelled antigen is applied. Labelled and unlabelled antigens compete with each other for the antibodies' binding sites. The greater the amount of test antigen that is present, the less labelled antigen will bind to the antibody. Calibration curves using known quantities of unlabelled antigen are established. The technique is often used for assaying hormones.

Radioimmunosorbent Test (RIST) is a competition RIA test as used to detect IgE (the antigen), in which test IgE is competed with labelled IgE on plates sensitized with anti-IgE.

Capture radioimmunoassays use antigen or antibody bound to the solid phase to capture molecules from the test solution, which are then detected with radiolabelled reagents. For example, solid phase anti-IgM captures IgM from the test solution, and the antigen-specific IgM is detected with a labelled antigen.

Sandwich radioimmunoassays are used to detect antibodies in systems where the test antibody acts as a bridge between solid phase unlabelled antigen and labelled antigen. The labelled antigen will only stick if specific antibody is present to bridge it to the solid phase.

Immunoradiometric Assay (IRMA) is a test for antigen in which excess specific labelled antibody is added to the test antigen. The test antigen binds and neutralizes some of the antibody - the remaining free antibody is removed by adding solid phase antigen. The labelled antibody still in solution is the proportion bound to the test antigen, and the radioactivity of the solution is proportional to the amount of test antigen.

Farr assay uses radiolabelled antigens to detect specific antibody. The test antibody is first mixed with the labelled antigen, then the antibodies are precipitated either using a specific precipitating reagent such as Staphylococci which have protein A in their cell walls, or by physicochemical precipitation with ammonium sulphate or polyethylene glycol. The amount of precipitated antigen is proportional to the amount of specific antibody. Some Farr assays use anti-Fc antibodies to precipitate the test antibody. These can be class or subclass specific to detect the amount of specific antibody of a particular isotype.

Enzyme Linked Immunosorbent Assay (ELISA) is used for detecting antibody. Antigen is adsorbed to a solid phase and test antibody is added as in the radioimmunoassay, but the ELISA ligand used to detect the antibody is an enzyme linked to a molecule specific for the bound antibody. Enzymes such as peroxidase and phosphatase are often used. In the final stage a chromogenic substrate is added, which generates a coloured end-product in the presence of the enzyme portion of the ligand. The optical density of this solution is measured after a defined period. This is proportional to the amount of enzyme, which in turn is related to the amount of test antibody. By comparison with RIA, this test has the advantage of stable reagents, but is usually less sensitive.

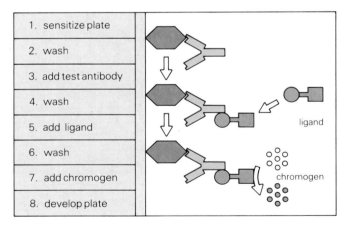

1. sensitize plate	
2. wash	
3. add test antibody	
4. wash	
5. add ligand	ligand
6. wash	
7. add chromogen	chromogen
8. develop plate	

Fig. 7.3 Enzyme linked immunosorbent assay.

Homogenous Enzyme Immunoassays (EMIT) are a group of assays to detect antigen using the antigen coupled to an enzyme in such a way that the activity of the enzyme is altered when the antigen binds to the antibody. The antigen/enzyme ligand then competes with the free (test) antigen for a binding site on a limiting amount of antibody, which is also present in the assay mixture (cf. competition radioimmunoassay). In this test it is not necessary to separate bound and unbound antigen.

Fluorescence Immunoassays (FIA) are analogous to radio immunassays, but substitute fluoresceinated reagents for the radiolabelled material. The method has the advantage that fluorescent reagents may be detected instantaneously, but problems can arise with the intrinsic fluorescence of the test material and also with the availability of suitable reagents. Some fluorescent reagents respond differently when they are bound to antibody and when free. In this case it is not necessary to separate bound and free fractions of the fluorescent reagent. Examples of this principle include:

Fluorescence quenching is the reduction of fluorescence emitted by an antibody (or antigen) when it forms a complex. For example, this occurs when a hapten, which absorbs radiation at 350nm, binds to an antibody. Normally, antibody illuminated at 280nm fluoresces at 350nm, but if the hapten is bound at the binding site some of the fluorescence is absorbed (quenched).

Fluorescence enhancement is the increased fluorescence produced by some haptens when bound to antibody. The energy is absorbed from the antibody and emitted with the wavelength characteristic of the hapten.

Fluorescence polarization. If polarized light is directed at a fluorescent molecule it is absorbed and emitted shortly afterwards, during which time the molecules move at random so that the fluorescent emission shows reduced polarization. If, however, the fluorescent molecule is bound to an antibody it has less rotational freedom and the polarization of the emission will be retained to a greater degree.

These properties of fluorescent reagents are used in the determination of antibody affinity and avidity. The determination of antibody affinity requires that the antigen and antibody react and reach a state of equilibrium. Since it is possible to determine the concentrations of bound and free fluorescent reagents without separating them, this is a great advantage because physical separation of the free and bound antigen may disturb the equilibrium conditions. Unfortunately suitable fluorescent reagents are only available for a few antigens and antibodies.

Equilibrium dialysis is the reference method for determining antibody affinity, in which a dialysable antigen or hapten and the test antibody are placed in chambers on opposite sides of a dialysis membrane. The system is left until the concentration of free antigen is the same on either side of the membrane (equilibrium), and then the solutions are sampled. The average affinity (K_o) is defined as the reciprocal of the free antigen concentration when half of the antibody's combining sites are occupied, so for IgG with two sites:

Affinity, $K_o = 1/[Ag_{free}]$

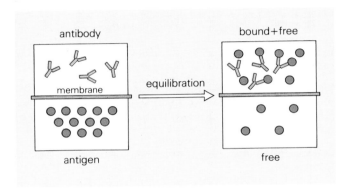

Fig.7.4 Equilibrium dialysis.

Scatchard equation is the general form for determining antibody affinity: $r/[Ag_{free}] = nK - rK$
where r is the number of antibody sites occupied (ie. the concentration of bound antigen), n is the antibody valency and K is the affinity constant. Plotting $r/[Ag_{free}]$ against r yields a curve of slope -K which intercepts the r axis at the point where all the antibody combining sites are occupied, that is n, the antibody valency.

Langmuir equation ($1/r = 1/nK . 1/[Ag_{free}] + 1/n$) is another formula which can be used to derive the affinity (K_o), and the number of available antibody binding sites (n), by plotting 1/r against $1/[Ag_{free}]$.

Sips equation ($\log r/(n-r) + a \log [Ag_{free}] + a \log K_o$) can be used to determine affinity (K_o) and the heterogeneity of a population of antibody molecules. Plotting $\log r/(n-r)$ against $\log[Ag_{free}]$ yields a line with slope = a, which is a measure of the heterogeneity of binding affinity.

Haemagglutination. This term covers a number of techniques for detecting antibodies, based on the agglutination of red blood cells. The antigen may either be a red cell antigen, or the antigen (sensitizing antigen) required can be chemically linked to the cell surface. For the test, the antibody is titrated in wells and the red cells added. If antibody to the red cell is present the cells are agglutinated and sink as a mat to the bottom of the well, but if it is absent they roll down the sloping sides of the well to form a pellet.

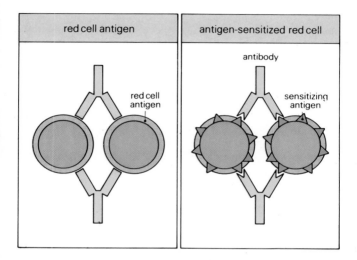

Fig.7.5 Haemagglutination test.

Direct and Indirect Coombs test are the original haemagglutination tests to detect antibodies to red cell antigens. The *direct Coombs test* identifies antibodies which are themselves capable of cross-linking the red cells. The *indirect Coombs test* detects antibodies which cannot crosslink the cells alone (eg. because there are too few antigens). This is acheived by the addition of a second layer anti-antibody.

Complement fixation test detects antibody (or antigen). Test antibody is mixed with the antigen and a small amount of active complement. If antibody is present complexes form and fix the complement, but if none is present active complement remains. Active complement is detected (if complexes did not form) by adding antibody sensitized red cells (EA), which lyse if complement is present. (To detect antigen, specific antibody is mixed with the test solution and complement.)

Precipitin reactions. When antigen and antibody react together near their equivalence point they often form cross-linked precipitates. If the reaction occurs in a supporting medium, such as an agar gel, the reactants form precipitin arcs, which can be used to identify antigens and antibodies in complex mixtures.

Immunodouble diffusion (Ouchterlony) is used to distinguish antigens in mixtures. The reactants are placed in holes punched in the gel, and diffuse together. The precipitin arcs may show one of three patterns. Where two arcs are fused this indicates identity between the antigens. If they form independently the antigens are not identical, and if the arcs are fused but with a spur, then the antigens are partially identical, but one antigen contains epitopes which the other lacks.

Countercurrent electrophoresis is a technique for detecting antigens or antibodies by forcing them to move together in an electric field. The technique is related to, but more sensitive than immunodouble diffusion.

Single Radial Immunodiffusion (SRID) (Mancini) is used to quantitate antibody. Test antibody is put in wells in an antigen containing gel, and diffuses out to form precipitin rings when it reaches equivalence. The area of the ring is proportional to antibody concentration. Antigen can be measured similarly using antibody containing gels.

Rocket electrophoresis is a modification of SRID in which antigens are quantitated by electrophoresing them through an antibody-containing gel, the pH of which is selected so that the antibodies are neutrally charged and immobile. The antigen moves towards the anode, forming a rocket shaped precipitin arc where the height of the rocket is proportional to antigen concentration.

Immunoelectrophoresis (IEP) is a technique in which mixtures of antigens are first separated in an electric field according to their charge, and are then precipitated with antiserum from a trough lying parallel to the separated antigens.

Crossed electrophoresis (Laurell) first separates antigens according to their charge in an electric field, in the first dimension. Then the antigens are electrophoresed into an antibody-containing gel at right angles to the first separation. In this case the area under the precipitin arcs is proportional to antigen concentration. This technique is useful for quantitating the different forms of an antigen, for example C3 and C3c, which share epitopes but have different charges.

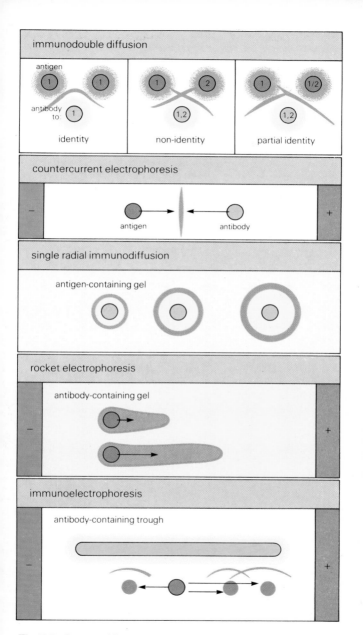

Fig.7.6 Agar gel immunoprecipitation techniques for identifying antigens and antibody.

Immunoabsorption is used to specifically remove particular antibodies from a solution, by the addition of a solid phase antigen immunoabsorbent.

Immunoabsorbents, that is, solid phase antigens or antibodies, include cells, chemically crosslinked antigen precipitates, and proteins coupled to solid supports.

Affinity chromatography is used to isolate pure antibodies. A column is prepared from antigen covalently coupled to an inert solid phase such as crosslinked dextran beads. The antibody-containing solution is run into the column in neutral buffer. Specific antibody binds to the antigen, while unbound antibody and other proteins are washed through. The specific antibody is eluted using a buffer which dissociates the antigen/antibody bond, that is, high or low pH or denaturing agents. By using antibody bound to the solid phase the technique can be used to isolate antigens.

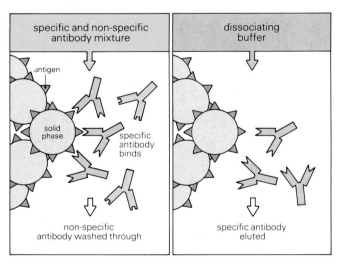

Fig.7.7 Affinity chromatography.

Affinity labelling is used to identify the amino acid residues in an antibody paratope, by the use of special haptens. These haptens have a highly reactive bond which is activated by illumination with UV light. When bound to the antibody these bonds attach to the nearest amino acids, that is, those forming the paratope. The antibody is then denatured and the location of the covalently coupled hapten determined.

Immunofluorescence is a general method for identifying antigens in tissue sections and on cells, or for identifying antibodies to them, as follows:

Direct immunofluorescence. The antibody is covalently coupled to a fluorescent molecule, such as fluorescein or rhodamine, which is then incubated with the cells or a frozen tissue section. The antibody binds to the antigen and this is then visualized by observing the material under a microscope with incident UV light.

Indirect immunofluorescence. In this technique the section is incubated with the test antibody, which is then visualized by the addition of a second layer fluorescent anti-antibody. The amplification produced by the second antibody increases the sensitivity of the assay, and by using class or subclass specific reagents particular isotypes can be identified in the test antibody. This technique is particularly valuable for identifying antibodies to tissue antigens, as illustrated below, where antibodies to a pancreatic islet of Langerhans in diabetic serum were identified by indirect immunofluorescence using a frozen section of pancreas.

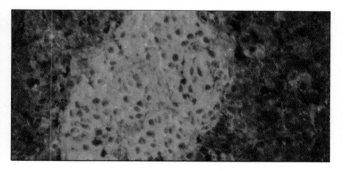

Fig.7.8 Islet cell autoantibodies demonstrated by immunofluorescence.

Capping occurs when antibodies bind and crosslink the surface antigens on a live cell. The antigens aggregate at one pole of the cell, appearing as a (fluorescent) cap. The cap is then internalized (capped off).

Cocapping is used to determine whether two different cell surface antigens are independent, in which case they form separate caps, with specific antibodies, or associated, when they form a single cap (cocap).

ISOLATION OF CELLS

Ficoll gradients are used to isolate cells of different densities. In particular they are used in the purification of lymphocytes. A diluted blood sample is layered onto the Ficoll and centrifuged. Since red blood cells and polymorphs are denser than Ficoll they sediment to the bottom, whilst the lymphocytes and some macrophages remain at the interface. Lymphocyte populations may be further depleted of macrophages by adherence, or by letting the phagocytes take up iron filings and then removing them with a magnet.

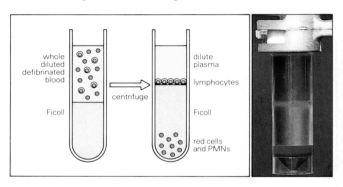

Fig.7.9 Separation of lymphocytes on a Ficoll isopaque gradient.

Adherence. Macrophages have the property of adhering to plastic, thus they may be removed from cell suspensions by plating on plastic dishes to which they adhere.

Panning uses plastic plates sensitized with antigen or antibody (cf. radioimmunoassay). Mixtures of cells are incubated on the plate and cells with receptors for the sensitizing agent bind to it. For example, cells with an antigen receptor will bind to an antigen-coated plate. The technique is often used to deplete cells of a specific subpopulation, but the bound cells can sometimes be recovered by chilling or digesting the plate with enzyme.

Nylon wool adherence is used to fractionate mouse lymphocytes. In physiological conditions, B cells and macrophages adhere to the nylon wool, while most T cells do not (some T cell blasts may also adhere). The B cells may be dissociated from the nylon wool by chilling and removing serum from the culture medium.

Rosetting is a method of isolating cells by allowing them to associate with red blood cells. Lymphocytes become surrounded (rosette) with the red cells and may then be isolated by sedimentation through Ficoll gradients.

E Rosettes. Human T cells have receptors for sheep erythrocytes (E) and so may be isolated by mixing with the sheep cells and separating the rosettes produced.

EA Rosettes. Cells which have Fc receptors for IgM or IgG can be isolated by mixing with red cells sensitized with antibody (EA) of the appropriate class. The antibody crosslinks the red cell to the Fc receptor and the rosettes are then isolated.

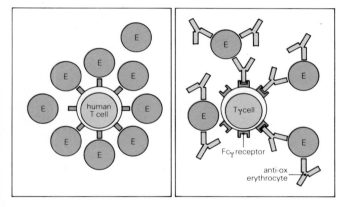

Fig.7.10 Isolation of cells by rosetting.

Antigen suicide is used to deplete those cells of a population which bind a particular antigen, by supplying them with highly radioactive antigen. This is taken up and kills the cell. A modification of this technique, to kill proliferating cells, is to add bromodeoxyuridine, which they incorporate. Illumination with UV light activates this metabolite to kill the cells.

Antibody/complement depletion. Particular cell populations can be lysed by treatment with specific antibody and complement, activated via the classical pathway.

Fluorescence Activated Cell Sorter (FACS) is a machine which can analyse the size and fluorescence intensity of single cells stained with specific fluorescent antibodies. The cells are then sorted according to these parameters with the exact conditions determined by the operator.

CLONES AND CELL LINES

Clone is a group of cells derived from a single original cell; they are therefore genetically identical.

Line is a group of cells grown in defined conditions from an initially heterogeneous population. Only occasionally will such a line be monoclonal.

Hybridomas are cells produced by the physical fusion of two different cells. Polyethylene glycol and Sendai virus are often used to effect the fusion. A hybridoma cell and its progeny contain some chromosomes from each fusion partner, although some others are usually lost.

Immune responses and antibody populations may be described according to the number of responding cells as:

Monoclonal, Oligoclonal, Polyclonal according to whether it is due to one, a few, or many clones.

Monoclonal antibodies are homogeneous antibodies produced by a single clone. They are usually made from hybridomas, which are prepared by fusing immunized mouse or rat spleen cells with a non-secretor myeloma using polyethylene glycol (PEG). The fusion mixture is plated out in HAT medium. HAT contains Hypoxanthine, Aminopterin and Thymidine. Aminopterin blocks a metabolic pathway which can be bypassed if hypoxanthine and thymidine are present, but the myeloma cells lack this bypass and consequently die in HAT medium. Spleen cells also die naturally in culture after 1 - 2 weeks, but fused cells survive since they have the immortality of the myeloma *and* the metabolic bypass of the spleen cells. Some of the fused cells secrete antibody, and the supernatants are tested in a specific assay. Wells which produce the desired antibody are then cloned.

Cloning by limiting dilution is a process in which a cell population is diluted sucessively and set up in culture so that there are wells containing only one cell. The progeny of this cell are grown on as a clone.

Cloning from soft agar is done by culturing a cell population in soft agar, which prevents the cells from moving. Colonies which develop around a single cell are removed by micromanipulation and cultured.

T cell lines are produced by culturing a population of primed T cells in the presence of antigen and/or interleukin 2. The antigen

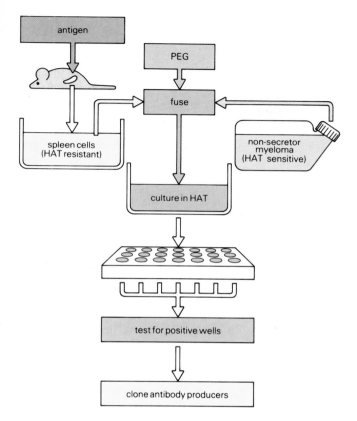

Fig.7.11 Monoclonal antibody production.

must be presented to the T cells in a recognizable form, usually on macrophages which have been treated to block their metabolism. T cell activity is assayed by antigen-specific proliferation.

Proliferation is usually measured by the uptake of radio-labelled metabolites required for DNA or RNA synthesis, such as ^{125}I-Uridine deoxyribose or ^{3}H-thymidine. The uptake of these metabolites is measured by harvesting the cells and counting the incorporated radioactivity.

Cell harvester is a machine which semi-automatically aspirates cell cultures, deposits them onto small paper filters and washes away free radioactive metabolites.

CELLULAR FUNCTIONS

Plaque Forming Cells (PFC) are antibody secreting cells measured in an assay where each secreting cell produces a clear zone of lysis (plaque) in a layer of antigen sensitized red blood cells (see Fig.7.13).

Indirect plaques measure antigen-specific IgG producers. The test lymphocytes are mixed and incubated with antigen-sensitized red cells (cf. haemagglutination). Antibody from specific B cells binds to the antigen on the red cells and the addition of antibody to IgG together with complement causes complement fixation on the red cells producing a plaque of lysed cells.

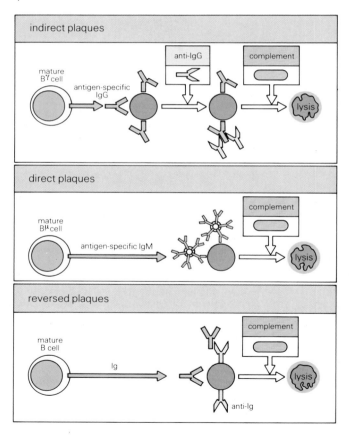

Fig.7.12 Plaque forming cell assays.

Direct plaques measure the numbers of antigen-specific IgM-producing cells. IgM is capable of fixing complement without the addition of a second layer antibody. Thus IgG and IgM producing cells can be quantitated separately.

Reversed plaques measure the total number of immunoglobulin producing cells (not just the antigen specific ones). Released antibody binds to red cells sensitised with anti-Ig (or protein A). This cell surface complex can now fix complement to produce a plaque.

Chromium release (cytotoxicity) assay is used to measure the activity of cytotoxic cells. The target cells are first mixed with radioactive ^{51}Cr which is taken up by viable cells. These are then incubated with the test leucocytes. If the test cells damage the targets the ^{51}Cr is released and can be measured in the supernatant.

Antibody-Dependent Cell Mediated Cytotoxicity (ADCC) is produced by K cells and is often measured using chicken erythrocytes as the labelled target in the presence of erythrocyte specific antibody.

Mixed Lymphocyte Target Interaction (MLTI) is a modified one-way mixed lymphocyte culture, to determine whether test lymphocytes recognize a particular target cell (often a tumour). The lymphocytes are mixed with inactivated targets, and the response measured by their uptake of radioactive metabolites.

NBT (Nitroblue Tetrazolium) reduction is a standard test for the oxidative burst in neutrophils.

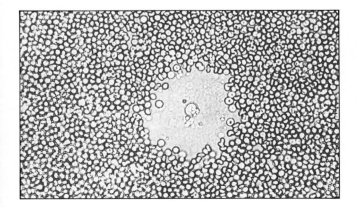

Fig.7.13 Antibody forming cell plaque.

PROTEIN FRACTIONATION AND ANALYSIS

Immunologists use many biochemical techniques. Some of those more commonly used are outlined below.

Gel filtration/permeation chromatography separates molecules on the basis of size by passing them through columns of microporous beads. Large molecules are excluded from the gel matrix and are eluted first.

Sucrose density gradient ultracentrifugation separates molecules on the basis of their size shape and density.

CsCl$_2$ gradient ultracentrifugation sediments molecules to a point where their density equals that of the CsCl$_2$ gradient, thus separating them on the basis of their buoyant density.

Ion exchange chromatography separates molecules on the basis of their charge. Charged molecules become adsorbed to the ion exchange medium and are sucessively eluted with increasing ion concentration.

Isoelectric focusing (IEF) analyses molecules according to their isoelectric point (pI), that is, the pH at which the molecule has an overall zero charge.

Spectrotype refers to the characteristic pattern given by a particular molecule separated by IEF. Even monoclonal antibodies produce several lines of different pI, due to post synthetic modifications.

SDS PAGE (Sodium Dodecyl Sulphate Polyacrylamide Gel Electrophoresis) is a technique to analyse polypeptides according to their size. Proteins treated with SDS become strongly negatively charged and are then electrophoresed through a polyacrylamide gel which acts as a molecular sieve. Since larger peptides bind more SDS, different peptides have similar charge/size ratios and the rate at which they pass through the gel is dependent solely on their size. Smaller molecules are retarded to a lesser degree and migrate fastest.

O'Farrell two dimensional gel separates proteins in an IEF gel in the first dimension and on an SDS polyacrylamide gel in the second, so as to give both the pI and size of the molecules.

Blotting is the technique of transferring proteins separated in polyacrylamide gels onto a reactive 'paper' (eg. nitrocellulose). Blotted proteins are more readily identified by immunochemical techniques than in the original gels.

Immunoblotting is used to identify blotted proteins by incubating the blot with radiolabelled antibody (or antigen). The antibody binds to antigens on the blot whose location is detected by autoradiography. The bound antibody can also be detected by using a second layer radiolabelled anti-antibody, or enzyme conjugated antibody (cf. radioimmunoassay and ELISA).

Autoradiography is used to locate radiolabelled materials present in gels or blots, where the test material is directly overlaid with a sheet of film.

Notes